Shrotri's

Surgical Principles in
Obstetrics and
Gynaecology

Eighth Edition

Shrotri's

Surgical Principles in
Obstetrics and
Gynaecology

Eighth Edition

Nishikant Shrotri MD, DGO
Consultant Obstetrician and Gynaecologist

Aparna Shrotri MD, DGO
Ex-Professor, Obstetrics and Gynaecology

CBS

CBS Publishers & Distributors Pvt Ltd

New Delhi • Bengaluru • Chennai • Kochi • Mumbai • Pune
Hyderabad • Kolkata • Nagpur • Patna • Vijayawada

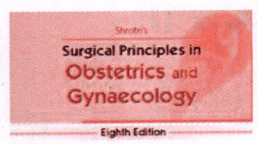

ISBN: 978-81-239-2255-3

Copyright © Authors

Eighth Edition: 2013

Reprint: 2015

First Edition: 1987

Published by Satish Kumar Jain and produced by Varun Jain for

CBS Publishers & Distributors Pvt Ltd

4819/XI Prahlad Street, 24 Ansari Road, Daryaganj, New Delhi 110 002, India.

Ph: 23289259, 23266861, 23266867   Website: www.cbspd.com

Fax: 011-23243014.   e-mail: delhi@cbspd.com; cbspubs@airtelmail.in.

Corporate Office: 204 FIE, Industrial Area, Patparganj, Delhi 110 092

Ph: 4934 4934   Fax: 4934 4935   e-mail: publishing@cbspd.com; publicity@cbspd.com

Branches

- **Bengaluru:** Seema House 2975, 17th Cross, K.R. Road, Banasankari 2nd Stage, Bengaluru 560 070, Karnataka
  Ph: +91-80-26771678/79   Fax: +91-80-26771680   e-mail: bangalore@cbspd.com
- **Chennai:** 7, Subbaraya Street, Shenoy Nagar, Chennai 600 030, Tamil Nadu
  Ph: +91-44-42032115   Fax: +91-44-42032115   e-mail: chennai@cbspd.com
- **Kochi:** 36/14 Kalluvilakam, Lissie Hospital Road, Kochi 682 018, Kerala
  Ph: +91-484-4059061/65   Fax: +91-484-4059065   e-mail: kochi@cbspd.com
- **Mumbai:** 83-C, Dr E Moses Road, Worli, Mumbai-400018, Maharashtra
  Ph: +91-22-24902340/41   Fax: +91-22-24902342   e-mail: mumbai@cbspd.com
- **Pune:** Bhuruk Prestige, Sr. No. 52/12/2+1+3/2 Narhe, Haveli (Near Katraj-Dehu Road Bypass), Pune 411 041, Maharashtra
  Ph: +91-20-64704058/59, 32392277 Fax: +91-20-24300160   e-mail: pune@cbspd.com

Representatives

- **Hyderabad** 0-9885175004   • **Kolkata** 0-9831437309, 0-9051152362
- **Nagpur**   0-9021734563   • **Patna** 0-9334159340   • **Vijayawada** 0-9000660880

Printed at Magic International, Greater Noida, UP

to

the undergraduate students of obstetrics and gynaecology

Preface to Eighth Edition

This edition, like the previous ones, has been revised thoroughly by incorporating new, current knowledge and procedures and deleting the old and outdated material. In this edition, Dr (Mrs) Aparna Shrotri, who was so far helping with her able guidance, has kindly consented to participate in the capacity of coauthor. I am indeed thankful to her.

This edition of the book has come to the readers in a different two-colour presentation brought out by CBS Publishers & Distributors, New Delhi. It has taken a little longer to come out with the eighth edition of this book. This delay was due to my personal difficulties. All the illustrations have been completely redrawn to bring in clarity. The publisher has given us full cooperation for this edition. We are thankful to them for their patient support.

Nishikant Shrotri
Aparna Shrotri
40/1-A, Karve Road, Pune 411004
Maharashtra, India
nishikants@gmail.com

Preface to First Edition

We are living in the scientific era, wherein along with other scientific knowledge, medical knowledge is also expanding with unimaginable rate. The older concepts get gradually diluted with the addition of newer ones. With such a rapid turnover, the main principles get diluted in an unfathomable expansion of their applications.

In good old days there used to be individual teaching and direct rapport between the 'Guru' and the 'Shishya'. With ever-increasing number of students, such personal attention to the students is becoming more and more difficult.

Textbooks no doubt help the students in grasping the subject thoroughly, however, a rapid reference material is necessary, especially while appearing for the examinations or while managing a case in day-to-day practice.

Obstetrics, gynaecology and family welfare is a community-oriented subject having an appeal for every medical practitioner demanding his contribution for betterment of maternal and child health.

It was, therefore, felt necessary to have a concentrate of the main surgical principles in this subject for the use of undergraduate medical students. However, these excerpts cannot be substitute to the textbooks, nor to their hospital experience. This book can only serve the purpose of rapid systematic recapitulation at a glance.

This book is also expected to be useful for general practitioners, especially practising in peripheral areas, who generally do not undertake surgical management of the patients; but at the same time have to shoulder the responsibility of guiding the patients to such surgical management after explaining the nature and effect of it. This book does not aim to guide the practitioner to perform any operative procedure but tries to make him conversant with the different surgical procedures in this field.

I hope *Surgical Principles in Obstetrics and Gynaecology* will prove to be a reproducible knowledge-pack for the medical students and a ready-reference asset to the practitioners.

Nishikant Shrotri

Contents

Preface to Eighth Edition *vii*

Preface to First Edition *ix*

Section 1 Gynaecology 1

1. Endometrial Evaluation 3

2. Diagnosis of CIN and Carcinoma Cervix 12

3. Ablation (Physical Destruction) of Cervical Lesions 27

4. Tubal Infertility 33

5. Gynaecological Endoscopy 45

6. Hysterectomy 53

7. Genital Prolapse 65

8. Myomectomy 74

9. Ovarian Surgery 78

10. Urinary Incontinence 81

11. Congenital Malformations 95

Section 2 Obstetrics 99

12. Surgical Evacuation 101

13. Cervical Encerclage 105

14. Prenatal Diagnosis 112

15. Version 125

16. Episiotomy 130

17. Instrumental Vaginal Delivery   135

18. Caesarean Section   152

19. Obstetric Haemorrhage   169

20. Destructive Operations   175

21. Manual Removal of Placenta   180

Section 3 MTP and Family Planning   **183**

22. MTP Act   185

23. MTP Procedures   189

24. Natural Methods of Contraception   208

25. Barrier Contraception   213

26. Hormonal Contraception   222

27. Intrauterine Contraceptive Devices   238

28. Female Sterilization   253

29. Male Sterilization   268

Section 4 Drugs   **279**

30. Drugs in Obstetrics and Gynaecology   281

Section 5 Instruments in Obstetrics and Gynaecology   **335**

31. Opening Abdomen   337

32. Instruments   343

Index   363

Gynaecology

1. Endometrial Evaluation
2. Diagnosis of CIN and Carcinoma Cervix
3. Ablation (Physical Destruction) of Cervical Lesions
4. Tubal Infertility
5. Gynaecological Endoscopy
6. Hysterectomy
7. Genital Prolapse
8. Myomectomy
9. Ovarian Surgery
10. Urinary Incontinence
11. Congenital Malformations

Endometrial Evaluation

The endometrial study is indicated in women with menstrual abnormalities and for infertility evaluation.

The procedures for diagnosing endometrial diseases are histopathological studies of endometrial sample, hysteroscopy and microhysteroscopy.

The endocrinologic status of the woman, however, is indirectly studied from endometrial histology. Currently, sophisticated hormone assays are being used for this purpose.

Indications for Endometrial Curettage

Diagnostic

1. Menorrhagia
   - To exclude organic uterine pathology, e.g. carcinoma endometrium.
   - To differentiate between ovular and anovular dysfunctional uterine bleeding.
2. Postmenopausal bleeding
   - To exclude or diagnose endometrial carcinoma fractional curettage is performed.
3. Follow-up of vesicular mole
   - To exclude choriocarcinoma in cases of irregular bleeding
4. Suspicion of endometrial tuberculosis
5. Infertility
   - Diagnosis of endometrial tuberculosis
   - Detection of ovulation (USG is used for this purpose)

Therapeutic

6. *Menorrhagia:* Curettage helps to arrest the bleeding and can give relief in 30% cases.

ENDOMETRIAL BIOPSY

This procedure is used for obtaining a strip of endometrium for studying hormonal status of the woman. Such strip biopsy is appropriate to detect only the generalized changes, i.e. hormonal influences on the endometrium. Attempt to diagnose organic pathologies like endometrial tuberculosis or malignancy may be unsuccessful if the strip collected does not include the organic lesion.

DILATATION AND CURETTAGE

This operation comprises of dilatation of internal cervical os and curettage of the uterine cavity.

Indications for Dilatation Only

1. Spasmodic dysmenorrhoea
2. Drainage of pyometra
3. Initial step in Fothergill's operation
4. Initial step in operative hysteroscopy
5. For insertion of radiation source

Timing of Operation

Usually, curettage is performed premenstrually for detection of ovulation in infertile patients and for studying endocrine status of the woman. Currently, sonographic follicle monitoring is used for ovulation detection.

Curettage is performed on the first day of menstruation in women having irregular infrequent menses. It has an additional advantage of not disrupting possible pregnancy. Curettage may be performed on any day for therapeutic purpose to arrest the bleeding.

However, curettage is generally not performed in immediate postmenstrual phase. It carries the danger of intrauterine trauma and/or removing the basal endometrium, which is likely to create Aschermann's syndrome.

Contraindications

1. Pregnancy
2. Infection

Preoperative Preparations

- The patient is to be kept nil by mouth for 6 hours.
- Proper consent for the operation should be obtained.
- Patient's bladder should be emptied by voiding.

Anaesthesia

Usually the procedure is performed under short general anaesthesia; by IV Inj. Thiopental-Na, but also can be done under local anaesthesia, i.e. paracervical block by lignocaine 1%.

Instruments

- Sponge holding forceps
- Sim's or Auvard's speculum
- Anterior vaginal wall retractor
- Volsellum
- Playfair's probe
- Uterine sound
- A set of cervical dilators
- Curette

Steps of Operation

1. Patient's legs are tied in lithotomy position.
2. Perineum is painted and vagina cleaned thoroughly by antiseptic solutions
3. Suitable anaesthesia is given.
4. Vaginal examination is done under anaesthesia to confirm:
   - Position and size of uterus
   - Presence of any adnexal pathology
5. Sim's or Auvard's vaginal speculum is inserted in the vagina.
6. Anterior vaginal wall is retracted by anterior vaginal wall retractor to visualize cervix.
7. Anterior lip of the cervix is held by volsellum forceps.
8. Cervical canal is disinfected by iodine soaked cotton wound over Playfair's probe.

9. The length and the position of the uterus are assessed by uterine sound.
10. Depending upon the size of the curette the cervical canal is dilated; usually up to no. 8.
11. The cavity is curetted out with the help of sharp curette.

The curetted endometrium is collected over a piece of gauze, transferred to 10% formalin bulb and is sent for histopathological study. For studying the evidence of tuberculosis, it is sent in sterile bulb containing normal saline.

FRACTIONAL CURETTAGE

Indications

Abnormal uterine bleeding in perimenopausal or postmenopausal women.

Purpose

- To diagnose endometrial and endocervical malignancy.
- It helps in staging the endometrial carcinoma.
- It helps to decide the extent of surgery in endometrial carcinoma.

Steps of Operation

1. Endocervical curettage is performed: Sample 1
2. Length of uterine cavity is measured with uterine sound.
3. Internal cervical os is dilated.
4. Uterine cavity is curetted: Sample 2
5. The material is collected separately, labeled and sent for histopathological study.

As per current guidelines for management of endometrial carcinoma, the study of isthmial sample does not alter the management.

Hysteroscopically guided endometrial biopsy is superior to blind curettage and is replacing this procedure in modern setup.

The extent of surgery is to be decided according to the stage of malignancy and pathological grading.

Management Guidelines for Endometrial Cancer

Stage I disease needs surgicopathological staging at laparotomy to decide need for adjuvant radiotherapy which is required for:

- Grade III disease
- Myometrial invasion of >50%
- Unfavourable histopathology (papillary, clear cell, adenosquamous carcinoma)
- Positive pelvic nodes.

Complications of D and C

A. *Intraoperative Complications*

1. *Cervical lacerations:* When cervix needs forceful dilatation
2. *Failure to dilate the cervix:* If cervix is stenosed, dilatation may become impossible and the procedure might have to be abandoned or postponed. In such cases it is advisable to perform the procedure on the first day of the menses when the cervix becomes soft and yields very easily.
3. *Uterine perforation:* This can take place while using uterine sound, dilators or curette if these instruments are used with undue force or in wrong direction.

   Detection: There is sudden loss of resistance to the instrument. It enters inside for more than expected length. The sound confirms the diagnosis.

   Management: Most perforations can be managed conservatively with careful monitoring. Laparotomy is indicated only when there are signs of internal bleeding as explained in MTP complications.

B. *Late Complications*

Infection:

- Pre-existing infection may get flared up.
- Fresh infection may get introduced.

Infection is manifested by severe hypogastric pain, vaginal discharge, excessive bleeding and fever.

Infection is managed by antibiotics.

C. *Sequelae*

1. *Cervical incompetence due* to excessive dilatation of internal os of the cervix leading to midtrimester abortions or early preterm deliveries in future.

2. *Infertility* due to tubal block caused by infection

3. *Aschermann's syndrome:* Uterine synechia may form due to formation of adhesions between uterine walls. Curettage in the immediate postmenstural phase, repeated curettages or vigorous curettages may curette out the basal endometrium completely, resulting in secondary amenorrhoea, oligomenorrhoea, infertility or recurrent abortions.

   Diagnosis: By hysterosalpingography or hysteroscopy.

   Hysterosalpingography shows honeycomb appearance in the uterine cavity.

   Hysteroscopically, the adhesions can be broken hence hysteroscopy is diagnostic as well as can be therapeautic procedure. Subsequent reformation of adhesions is avoided by keeping the uterine walls apart by inserting an intrauterine contraceptive device or paediatric Foley's catheter. Oestrogens are given for building the endometrium.

Purpose of Dilatation and Curettage

A. *In Infertility*

- Exclusion or diagnosis of endometrial tuberculosis (detected in 5% of women).
- Detection of ovulation (Table 1.1).
- Diagnosis of luteal phase defect by endometrial dating as suggested by endometrial development lagging by more than 2 days (midluteal serum progesterone is used for this now).
- Detection of submucous fibroid by noting irregularity in the uterine cavity (USG and hysteroscopy are better diagnostic procedures). (For management of conditions Table 1.2.)

Table 1.1: Detection of ovulation by endometrial histology

Tissue	Proliferative	Secretory
Glands	• Surface epithelium gradually becomes taller	• Subnuclear vacuoles
	• No secretory activity	• Increased intracellular secretion pushing nuclei back to basement membrane
		• Discharge of secretions into gland lumen
		• Glands become crenated and corkscrew shaped
Stroma	• Initially compact- gradually becomes oedematous	• Most oedematous
Vessels	• Increasing vascularity with increasing coiling	• Coiled arteries become more spiral

Table 1.2: Further management based on histopathological diagnosis

A. Endometrial organic conditions

a. Tubercular endometritis	• Antitubercular chemotherapy
b. Carcinoma endometrium	• Management according to stage of malignancy and histologic type

B. Functional status

a. Proliferative endometrium	• Induction of ovulation in anovulatory infertility
	• Progestational therapy for dysfunctional uterine bleeding
b. Endometrial hyperplasia	• Vide—Table 1.3
c. Luteal phase defect	• Progestogens in pre-menstrual spotting
	• HCG/progesterone in infertility

B. *In Dysfunctional Uterine Bleeding*
- Excluding organic pathology like endometrial tuberculosis and malignancy.
- For differentiating dysfunctional uterine bleeding into ovular or anovular types, i.e. hormonal status of the woman.
- To diagnose endometrial hyperplasia.
- To arrest bleeding phase by curetting out endometrium completely.
- 30 to 40% women get relief from menorrhagia.

Endometrial Hyperplasia

Continuous estrogen stimulation in absence of cyclical progesterone results in endometrial hyperplasia which causes abnormal uterine bleeding
- May lead to endometrial cancer
- May be associated with estrogen producing ovarian tumors.

Architectural and Cytologic Features

- *Architecture:* Simple or complex (complexity and crowding of glandular epithelium). Unusual degree of epithelial proliferative activity, pseudostratification or actual stratification.
- *Cytologic atypia:* Large nucleus, variable size and shape, lost polarity, increased nuclear cytoplasmic ratio, prominent nucleoli.

Classification

- Simple or complex architecture
- With or without cytologic atypia.

Malignant Potential of Different Types (Table 1.3)

- Simple: 1%
- Complex: 3%
- Simple with atypia: 8%
- Complex with cellular atypia: 29%

Progestin therapy (medroxyprogesterone acetate 10–20 mg daily) can reverse endometrial hyperplasia without atypia.

Table 1.3: Endometrial hyperplasia

Hyperplasia	HPE	Risk of malignancy	Management
Simple (cystoglandular)	• Glands dilated and cystic • Stroma compact	1%	• Young patients: Cyclical progestogen therapy • Elderly patients and family completed: Hysterectomy
Complex	• Extreme proliferation of glands resulting in obliteration of intervening stroma—back to back crowding	3%	• Family completed: Hysterectomy • Young patients desirous of pregnancy: Cyclical progestogen
Simple atypical	• Cells show varying degrees of atypia • Unusual degree of epithelial proliferative activity	8%	Hysterectomy advised as possibility of associated endometrial cancer or progression to endometrial cancer is high
Complex atypical	• Cells show atypia and are disorderly arranged	29%	Immediate hysterectomy with bilateral salpingo-oophorectomy

2

Diagnosis of CIN and Carcinoma Cervix

Carcinoma of cervix is still the commonest genital tract malignancy amongst the Indian female population. Unfortunately it is diagnosed quite late and causes many deaths.

There is a spectrum of premalignant conditions of cervix termed as **cervical intraepithelial neoplasia** or **CIN** which are of three types. Earlier these conditions were called as dysplasia. These lesions gradually progress to invasive malignancy over a period of many years.

CERVICAL INTRAEPITHELIAL NEOPLASIA (CIN)

- **CIN I:** Undifferentiated cells confined to the lower 1/3 of the epithelium (previously known as **mild dysplasia**)
- **CIN II:** Undifferentiated cells confined to the basal 2/3 of the epithelium **(moderate dysplasia).**
- **CIN III:** Involves greater than 2/3 of the epithelium, **(severe dysplasia)** and may involve the full thickness. The lesion involving full thickness of epithelium is referred to as **cervical carcinoma in situ (CIS)**/adenocarcinoma in situ where the stratification is lost but the basement membrane is intact and there is **no** stromal invasion.

CIN I can show spontaneous regression in 60–85% within 2 years. **CIN II/III** lesions progress to CIS in 20% and to invasive cancer in 5%, hence are more significant lesions.

These premalignant conditions can be diagnosed by various techniques such as:

- Exfoliative cytology
- HPV testing
- Colposcopy and colpomicroscopy
- Histopathological studies of biopsy specimens

Cervical cytology and HPV testing are screening procedures.

Abnormal results of screening tests need further evaluation by colposcopy and abnormal colposcopic findings require directed biopsy to identify presence and degree of CIN.

With these evaluative techniques, premalignant lesions of the cervix are detected early, which can be treated by different **ablative** or **excisional** therapeutic modalities; thus eliminating the possibility of subsequent development of invasive carcinoma of cervix.

EXFOLIATIVE CYTOLOGY

It is the study of pathological changes in exfoliated cells from genital tract.

This valuable diagnostic tool was first introduced into clinical practice by Papanicolaou and Traut, and was used mainly as a **screening test** for early detection of genital malignancy.

This technique is currently used for screening asymptomatic women for genital malignancies, especially for carcinoma of cervix.

Principle: Malignant cells get exfoliated in large numbers in comparison to normal cells which require more force for their separation. Smears are made from these cells for cytological studies.

Obtaining Material for Cytological Smears

a. *Cervical Scrape*

This is also known as surface biopsy. It is done by using Ayre's spatula. A cytobrush or moistened cotton tipped applicator can also be used in place of Ayre's spatula.

Ayre's spatula is rotated through 360° over the ectocervix and the material is spread on a clean glass slide.

Advantages
- Cells are fresh, as they are not shed.
- Detection of carcinoma cervix is easy and more accurate as the squamocolumnar junction is scraped.

Disadvantage
Cells from vagina and endometrium cannot be visualized.

b. Aspiration of Endocervical Canal and Uterine Cavity

Lesions of endocervix and endometrial cavity are diagnosed better as there is no contamination with other cells.

c. Aspiration from Posterior Fornix

Advantage: Cells from the complete genital tract get shed into posterior fornix.

Disadvantages

- Cells are few in number; hence malignancy is likely to be missed. Cells are devitalised.
- Unsuitable for woman with prolapse. Not recommended for screening of cancer cervix.

Vaginal smear should be deferred if:

- Vaginal bleeding
- Active infection
- Vaginal examination performed within previous 24 hours
- Vaginal antiseptics used.

Fixing and Staining of Smears

The smears are fixed immediately in mixture of equal quantities of alcohol 95% and ether. The smear is stained with Papanicolaou staining technique. The cellular details are studied carefully.

Alternatively liquid based cytology technique can be used. This reduces number of inadequate smears needing repeat smears. Sensitivity is improved and the sample can be used for reflex HPV testing. However, this technique is more expensive and false positive results are increased.

Cellular Criteria Suggesting Malignancy

a. Increased nuclear-cytoplasmic ratio
b. Hyperchromatism with coarsely granular chromatin network
c. Cells vary in size and shape
d. Nuclear changes:
   - Gross enlargement of nucleus
   - Irregular nuclear outline

- Multinucleation
- Reduplication of nucleoli
- Atypical mitosis

Bethesda System (2001)

- *Statement of adequacy:* Satisfactory for evaluation
- Negative for intraepithelial lesion/epithelial cell abnormality
- *Organisms:* Trichomonas, candida, bacterial vaginoses, actinomyces sp., HSV
- *Epithelial cells:* Squamous, glandular
- *Abnormal squamous cells (ASC):*
  - ASC-US: Unknown significance
  - ASC-H: High-grade lesions need to be excluded
- *LSIL:* Low-grade squamous intraepithelial lesions
- *HCIL:* High-grade squamous intraepithelial lesions
- Cancer
- *AGC:* Abnormal glandular cells

Cytology Screening

- Start 21 yrs or within 3 yrs of sexual debut
- Up to 30 yrs yearly (2 yearly by liquid base cytology) above 30 yrs without any risk factor 2–3 yearly
- Above 30 yrs: Smear and HPV DNA both negative assuring
- 3 yearly if 3 annual smears are normal

Role of Cytology

Cytology should be used for screening asymptomatic women. Symptomatic patients should be subjected to biopsy.

Main advantage of mass screening is the detection of cervical intraepithelial neoplasia (CIN), especially those that are known to progress towards invasive malignancy of cervix. Eradication of these lesions by ablative or excisional procedures, (cryosurgery, laser, LEEP, conization or hysterectomy) definitely reduces the occurrence of invasive carcinoma of cervix.

Limitations of Cytology
- Expensive method
- High technical expertise is required
- Not diagnostic by itself and histopathological confirmation of diagnosis by biopsy is necessary
- Confusing interpretation during pregnancy
- Limited accuracy–fair percentage of false negative and false positive smears
- Error in diagnosis is considerably high in cases of endometrial carcinoma.

Other Uses of Cytology
a. Assessment of endocrine status of a woman
   - Presumptive evidence of ovulation
   - Investigation in cases of amenorrhoea
   - Rational basis for substitution therapy with oestrogen or progesterone
   Smear is prepared from scraping of lateral vaginal wall. Not used currently as diagnostic endocrine assays are available.
b. *Peritoneal fluid cytology:* Blood stained fluid with malignant cells helps in diagnosis of carcinoma ovary.

COLPOSCOPY

Colpocsopy is useful to evaluate the changes in the terminal vascular network of the cervix. Cytology evaluates the morphological changes in the exfoliated cells of the genital tract.

Instrument

The colposcope is a stereoscopic microscope through which the cervix may be visualised in bright light with 6X to 40X magnification. However, routinely, 46X magnification is used.

Procedure

1. Self-retaining speculum is inserted in vagina to visualise cervix. Mucus is removed from the cervix.
2. Cervical surface is moistened with normal saline.

3. Optimal contrast of the vessels is acheived by insertion of green filter.
4. Acetic acid 4% is applied to the cervix, which coagulates the mucus and removes intracelluar water temporarily.

Stereoscopic evaluation of the transformation zone is done. Transformation zone extends between the original squamo-columnar junction and the physiological squamocolumnar junction, i.e. zone between metaplastic epithelium and columnar epithelium. It has been shown that cervical metaplasia develops almost exclusively within the transformation zone.

Immature squamous epithelium, epithelium with dysplasia or epithilial cells in carcinoma in situ have high nuclear mitotic activity. In such areas of high nuclear density, the epithelium becomes white on application of acetic acid.

To predict the type of histopathological changes, evaluation of vascular pattern, intercapillary distance, surface contour, colour tone and clarity of demarcation of focal lesion is necessary.

1. *Vascular pattern:* Alterations in the vascular pattern is the earliest change.
2. Intercapillary distance is increased.
3. *Surface contour:* Uneven or elevated
4. *Colour tone:* Marked changes from deep red to white before and after the acetic acid test indicates more serious histological lesion.
5. Border between the lesion and adjacent normal tissue.
   - Sharp-bordered lesions distinctly demarcated from adjacent epithelium in CIN.
   - Diffuse border is suggestive of inflammation.
6. Whenever, there are unsatisfactory colposcopic findings, other diagnostic methods like endocervical curettage or conization are required.

Value of Colposcopy

a. Accurate differentiation between invasive and noninvasive lesions is possible.
b. Differentiation between inflammatory atypia and neoplasia is possible.

It is ideal for evaluation of pregnant women with abnormal cytology. Physiological eversion of pregnant cervix helps good visualisation of squamocolumnar junction.

Colposcopy is used in vaginal microbicide research to assess the product induced inflammation.

Colposcopy in Therapy

a. Laser vapourization of cervix is performed under colposcopic guidance.
b. Extent of conization excision can be decided colposcopically.

Colposcopic Findings

Group 1	Original epithelium–columnar or native squamous
Group 2	Typical transformation zone (physiological metaplasia)
Group 3	Atypical transformation zone (atypical metaplasia) • White epithelium • Leukoplakia • Atypical blood vessels–mosaic, punctation
Group 4	a. Suspected overt cancer b. Overt cancer
Group 5	*Miscellaneous:* Inflammatory changes, atrophic epithelium, true erosion, condyloma, polyp, etc.
Unsatisfactory	Squamocolumner junction cannot be visualised properly.

Limitations of Colposcopy

a. Squamocolumnar junction within the cervical canal cannot be completely visualized, e.g. in postmenopausal women.
b. Cervix treated by diathermy, cryocautery, laser or conization has got drastically altered areas of metaplasia.
c. Glandular lesions like adenocarcinoma in situ or frank adenocarcinoma cannot be excluded with certainty by colposcopy and requires conization.

CERVICAL BIOPSY

This is a procedure for obtaining a piece of cervical tissue for histopathological study for the diagnosis of cervical malignancy.

Indications

1. *Clinical suspicion of cervical malignancy:*
   - Postcoital bleeding
   - Postmenopausal bleeding
   - Intermenstrual bleeding
   - Excessive vaginal discharge
   - Ulcer, nodule, growth or indurated plaque on the cervix which bleeds on touch
   - Unhealthy cervix
2. Abnormal cytological smear from cervix where colposcopic appearance is suggestive of malignancy.

Types of Cervical Biopsies

1. *Punch biopsy:* Obtained by cervical biopsy punch.
2. *Wedge biopsy:* A wedge of tissue from the selected site of the cervix is taken by bistoury knief.
3. *Four quadrant biopsy:* The biopsies are taken from the four quadrants of cervix along with endocervical curettage for improving the accuracy of the diagnosis.
4. Directed biopsy
5. Loop electrosurgical excision procedure (LEEP)
6. Cone biopsy
   Surface biopsy: Cytological smear, no tissue obtained.

DIRECTED BIOPSY

- **Schiller's test: Visual inspection of cervix with Lugol's iodine (VILI).** The cervix is painted with Gram's solution (one part of iodine + two parts of potassium iodide + 300 parts of water). The mature cells of well-oestrogenised squamous epithelium of the cervix and vagina contain abundant glycogen. On application of Lugol's iodine, it turns deep mahogany brown while nonglycogenated areas remain unstained. Rapidly dividing carcinomatous cells contain less glycogen and thus remain unstained. It is from this **Schiller light** area the biopsy is taken.

- **Visual inspection of cervix with acetic acid (VIA):** The cervix is painted by 3–4% acetic acid, which coagulates the nuclear proteins and gives the tissue white appearance. Such aceto-white area is selected for biopsy.
- **Toluidine blue test:** The cervix is painted by toluidine blue 1% and then washed with acetic acid 1%. Both DNA of nuclei and RNA of cytoplasm fix toluidine blue. The intensity of the staining depends upon the amount of chromatin, size of nuclei in the cell and number of nuclei per unit area of epithelium. Therefore, the biopsy is taken from stained area.
- **Colposcopy:** Vide supra.
- **Colpomicroscopy:** Colposcope giving a magnification up to 200X is used. The cervical epithelium is stained by hematoxyline and visualised through colpomicroscope to select the site for biopsy.

Timing of Surgery

Preferably postmenstrual phase of the cycle.

Instruments

- General instruments for vaginal surgery
- Cervical biopsy punch or Allis forceps and bistoury (no. 11) with handle.

Steps of Operation

1. Cervix is visualised and held with volsellum forceps.
2. The biopsy site should include the squamocolumnar junction near the suspicious area. Biopsy is taken with the help of cervical biopsy punch.

   Alternatively

   Biopsy site is held firmly with Allis forceps and a wedge shaped biopsy is taken with the help of bistoury from the edge of the growth or lesion.

3. The amount of bleeding from the site of biopsy is noted. If cosiderable bleeding is seen, it can be controlled by:
   - Tight packing of vagina for 6 hours
   - Catgut stitch
   - Cauterization of the site of bleeding
4. The cervical tissue is sent to the laboratory in 10% formaline for histopathological study.

Complications

1. *Primary haemorrhage:* Vide supra
2. *Infection:* Treated by suitable antibiotics
3. *Secondary haemorrhage:* Usually this can be managed by tight vaginal packing. Secondary haemorrhage may be due to infection, which requires antibiotics.

Information Obtained by Cervical Biopsy

1. Diagnosis of precancerous lesions, CIN 1, 2, 3
2. Confirms or excludes cervical malignancy
3. Indicates cellular type of malignancy
   Squamous cell carcinoma/adenocarcinoma
4. Information regarding histopathological grading
   Degree of anaplasia that indicates prognosis
5. Depth of invasion

Loop Electrosurgical Excision Procedure (LEEP)

This procedure is one of the most commonly used approaches to treat high grade cervical dysplasia (CIN II/III). It is performed with the help of low voltage diathermy. This technique can be used in an office setting under colposcopic guidance, under local anaesthesia. It is an alternative to cone biopsy.

Loop dimensions can vary in width and depth. The cervical transformation zone and lesion are excised to an adequate depth, which in most cases is at least 8 mm, and extending 4 to 5 mm beyond the lesion.

Therapeutic success up to 1 year is 95–97%.

Complications

- Vaginal bleeding and discharge for 2 weeks
- Secondary haemorrhage occasionally
- Increased risk of preterm delivery, LBW infants, preterm PROM in subsequent pregnancy.

CONE BIOPSY

Cone biopsy (Fig. 2.1) or conization of cervix is a procedure in which a conical tissue of the cervix including entire squamo-columnar junction is removed; which can be diagnostic as well as therapeutic.

The cone can be shallow or deep. The extent of the cone is decided by the extent of the lesion, whether the lesion is completely visible and whether the family is complete.

The size of the cone depends upon the extent of the lesion. In general, broader the base of the lesion, spread of the lesion in the cervical canal is likely to be of lesser extent. Hence, with appreciable ectocervical component of the lesion, the cone can be broad and shallow. With a small ectocervical lesion, its major part is likely to be extending in the cervical canal; hence, a narrow but elongated cone is removed.

Indications

1. Abnormal cytological smear from the cervix where
   - Colposcope is not available.
   - Transformation zone is not completely visible on colposcopy.
2. Lesions extending into the cervical canal outside the range of colposcope.
3. Target biopsy showing CIN III (severe dysplasia/carcinoma in situ) or microinvasive lesion–to exclude deeper invasion, conization is necessary.
4. Abnormal findings on endocervical curettage.
5. Poor correlation between cytology, colposcopy and histopathology of a clinical lesion necessitate conization for proper diagnosis, e.g. colposcopically the lesion is arousing

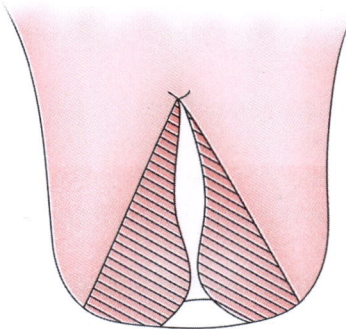

Fig. 2.1: Cone biopsy

the suspicion of invasive disease but the biopsy shows less severe disease.

Anaesthesia

Low spinal, general anaesthesia or paracervical block.

Steps

1. Visualisation and holding of cervix.
2. Base of the cone is demarcated by painting the cervix with iodine; or by colposcopy. To locate the normal anatomical position of the cervix, a stitch is taken at 12 O'clock position. This helps the pathologist while taking multiple sections.
3. The tissue of the base of the cone is held firm by one or more Allis forceps and the cone converging towards the internal os is cut by bistoury.
4. The raw area of the cervix can be covered by vaginal flaps by putting Sturmdorff suture (vide Fothergill's operation). However, this makes the further cytological follow-up of the residual lesion difficult hence not done.
5. Bleeding during the procedure can be minimised by lateral cervical sutures or intracervical injection of adrenaline.
6. A tight pack is kept in the cervical canal to prevent the bleeding which is removed after 6 to 24 hours.
7. Cold knife or laser can be used for conization.

Complications

1. *Bleeding:* Primary or secondary
2. Infection
3. Injury to the adjacent structures
4. *Cervical incompetence:* As deep conization may damage the circular muscle fibers of the internal os.
5. *Infertility:* May be the result of cervical stenosis or altered cervical mucus.
6. Cervical dystocia may result due to fibrosis and complicate labour.

Follow-Up

- Initial follow-up is after 2 months to note the healing.
- Thereafter, six monthly follow-up is performed for two years; and anually later.
- Follow-up consists of cytology, colposcopy and target biopsy when indicated.

Post Conization Hysterectomy

If hysterectomy is indicated urgently, it may be undertaken within 48–72 hours. Ideally it should be deferred for six weeks so that the congestion and fibrosis is minimal.

Management Guidelines

- If cone margin is free from neoplastic lesion and no invasive carcinoma is detected, the conization itself will prove to be therapeutic and curative.

  Still regular follow-up of these cases by cervical cytological smears is necessary.
- If cone margin shows cervical intraepithelial neoplasia III or microinvasion, hysterectomy with removal of cuff of vagina is indicated.
- If cone reveals invasive carcinoma; then radical hysterectomy or radiotherapy, as per the choice is indicated.

Significance of Abnormal Cervical Smear and Suggested Management

- *ASC-US:* CIN II/III in 3–5%. Any one of the three approaches can be selected
  - Repeat smear at 6 and 12 months, colposcopy if smear is abnormal
  - Immediate colposcopy
  - HPV DNA testing: If positive, colposcopy is done
- *ASC-H:* CIN II/III >30%. Colposcopy should be done. If colposcopy does not detect CIN II/III, HPV DNA testing at 12 months or cytologic testing at 6 and 12 months is advised.
- *LSIL:* CIN II/III 15–30%, hence colposcopy should be done.
- *HCIL:* CIN II/III 70%, invasive cancer 1–2% hence immediate colposcopy and LEEP is recommended. Follow-up cytology and colposcopy should be done in 4–6 months.
- *Atypical glandular cells:* Risk of adenocarcinoma in situ or invasive cancer is high. Colposcopy and endocervical curettage is recommended. Cone biopsy is needed to exclude more advanced lesions.

Table 2.1: Classification of cervical cytology smear by different methods

Bethesda (2001)	Dysplasia	CIN	Pap
Within normal limits	Normal	Negative	I
Infection (specify organism)	Inflammation		II
Reactive and reparative changes			
Squamous cell abnormalities	Squamous atypia		
Atypical squamous cells	HPV atypia		
i. ASC-US			
ii. ASC-H			
Low-grade squamous intraepithelial lesion (LSIL)	Mild	CIN I	
High-grade squamous intraepithelial lesion (HCIL)	Moderate dysplasia	CIN II	III
	Severe dysplasia Carcinoma in situ	CIN III	IV
Squamous cell carcinoma	Invasive cancer	Invasive cancer	V

In past, cervical cytology smears were graded (I, II, III, IV, V) as suggested by papanicolaou. Later, they were classified as mild, moderate and severe dysplasia. The correlation of these terminologies with currenty followed Bethesda system and the histopathological diagnosis as CIN I, II, III is shown in Table 2.1.

ADENOCARCINOMA OF ENDOCERVIX

Currently, the incidence of adenocarcinoma of the endocervix is found to be increasing. Adenocarcinoma in situ is its precursor. Entire endocervical canal is at risk. The lesions can be located above the transformation zone. A small lesion can be missed by cytology or cervical biopsy. Cytobrush for obtaining samples and endocervical curettage may improve the detection rate. However, conization is necessary to detect small lesions. The pyramidal cone may prove to be inadequate for complete evaluation of endocervical canal. A somewhat cylindrical cone may improve the accuracy of diagnosis.

3

Ablation (Physical Destruction) of Cervical Lesions

Indications

Cervical intraepithelial neoplasia of various grades: CIN I and CIN II diagnosed on colposcopically directed biopsy provided:

- Squamocolumnar junction is fully visible.
- Endocervical curettage is negative.
- Patient can be relied upon for regular follow-up.
- Invasive malignancy is thoroughly excluded.

These premalignant lesions of the cervix can be treated by various methods and invasive carcinoma of the uterine cervix can be prevented.

Cervical ectopy: Often called as cervical erosion is not a precancerous condition; but it is necessary to exclude the presence of possible neoplastic lesion by doing cervical cytological study.

Oestrogen dependent erosion observed during pregnancy or oral contraceptive therapy needs no intervention.

Methods

1. Electrocautery
2. Electrocoaguation diathermy
3. Cryotherapy
4. Laser vapourization
5. *Chemical cauterization:* The eroded cervical tissue is chemically destroyed by silver nitrate.

Ablation is appropriate when

- No microinvasion or invasion is suspected by cytology, colposcopy, endocervical curettage and biopsy

- Lesion is on the ectocervix and is visible entirely
- No involvement of endocervix.

Time of Procedure

- Postmenstrual phase of cycle; so that sufficient time is given for the healing before next menstrual period starts; thus avoiding the chances of infection.
- Early pregnancy ruled out.

Contraindications

- Pregnancy
- Presence of active infection
- Suspicion of malignancy.

CAUTERIZATION

1. Electrocautery

- OPD procedure, can be performed without anaesthesia by cautery machine
- Cervical lesion is cauterized radially by electrically preheated probes
- Depth of destruction up to 2 mm from the surface
- Less effective in comparison to other methods for treating CIN lesions.

2. Electrocoagulation Diathermy

- Performed in operation theatre under general anaesthesia
- Lesion is cauterized by flow of current when touched with probe of diathermy cautery
- More extensive and thorough destruction of lesion possible
- Depth of tissue destruction can be controlled
- Lesion, deep within glands may escape destruction
- In addition to the focal lesion, the transformation zone and columnar epithelium in the lower canal is also destroyed
- Follow-up by exfoliative cytology and colposcopy necessary.

Post-cauterization Instructions

- Due to sloughing of cauterized tissue, usually there is excessive vaginal discharge for a period of about two weeks. At times, this discharge may be blood stained.
- Abstinence till next period is over.
- Follow-up internal examination after the next menstrual period is necessary to note the healing of cauterized area.

Complications

- Extensive cauterization may lead to fibrosis of cervix and stenosis of cervical canal. Rarely, this may lead to cryptomenorrhoea.
- Incomplete cauterization as revealed by :
  a. Persistence of symptoms
  b. Presence of lesion on follow-up examination.
  It is treated by recauterization.

CRYOTHERAPY

Destruction of cervical lesions by cryosurgery is done by refrigeration of the tissues. The commonly used freezing agent is nitrous oxide. It is delivered to the lesion through a gun-type unit with interchangeable probes to bring about the freezing of tissues.

Nitrous oxide is applied either continuously or through cycles of 3 minutes freezing followed by 5 minutes thawing. The refrigerant is circulated until the iceball extends at least 5 mm beyond the edge of the lesion.

Heat exchange occurs at the probe, which lies at the surface of the tissue to be frozen. Heat is withdrawn by extreme low temperature created at the cryogun to form ice in the tissue. Cell death is effected primarily by dehydration, which increases the intracellular solute concentration and destroys protein. Rapid freezing and slow thawing is most lethal to the tissues. Repeated cycles of freezing-thawing enhance the tissue destruction.

Advantages
- Office procedure–no anaesthesia required
- No risk of fibrosis or stenosis
- No adverse effect on reproductive capacity
- Economical

Procedure

1. Exposing the cervix and removing the mucous plug by mucolytic agent (acetic acid 3%).
2. Cervical probe is passed which approximates anatomical configuration of the cervix and maximally covers the unhealthy area for selection. Then the probe is attached to the cryounit.
3. In cases of large lesions, the lesion is divided into smaller subdivisions which are frozen individually.
4. After positioning the probe, refrigerant is circulated.
5. Crystallization appears first at the tip of the probe, which spreads rapidly laterally onto the tissue.
6. Duration of freezing is around 2–5 minutes.
7. The edge of the iceball formed should extend 5–6 mm onto the normal appearing epithelium.
8. After the treatment, the probe is defrosted and disengaged from the cervix.

Postoperative

- Clear watery vaginal discharge for 2–3 weeks. Mucoid discharge for 1–2 weeks.
- Mild discomforting cramps in the lower abdomen for a couple of days.

Instructions to the Patient

- Abstinence for 3 weeks.
- Not to use any tampons.
- Follow-up after 4 weeks.
- Healing is usually complete within 6–8 weeks.

Results

- Depth of destruction up to 10 mm, tissue destruction up to 2–5 mm.
- *Failure to cure CIN lesions:* 10% with single freezing, 5% after refreezing
- *Criteria of cure for CIN:* Three consecutive cytological smears should be negative along with negative endocervical curettage.
- Failures are related to large lesion, CIN III, positive endocervical curettage, endocervical gland involvement.
- Suitable for CIN I/II, small lesion, ectocervical location only, negative ECC, no edocervical gland involvement on biopsy.

CO_2 LASER THERAPY

Light Amplification by Stimulated Emission of Radiation

Laser is a device for converting some form of energy, such as heat, light or electricity into radiant energy of special kind at one or more discrete wavelengths.

The radiation emitted by all lasers has three special qualities:

- *Coherent:* All the waves are exactly in phase with each other, in both space and time.
- *Collimated:* The rays are parallel to each other.
- *Monochromatic:* All the waves are of same wavelength.

The most efficient laser is CO_2 laser. It converts about 15% of its energy into coherent output radiation.

For treating the cervical lesion, the laser is attached to a colposcope. The depth of destruction is controlled by regulating the power density and the time.

Laser destroys tissue by vaporizing the intracellular fluid at the speed of light. A lot of smoke is produced in this procedure. Best results are obtained when tissue destruction is 5–7 mm. Incomplete destruction leads to persistence of lesion.

Advantages

- *Side effects are very few:* Postoperative discharge and bleeding are slight or nil.

- Vaporized site heals quickly and cleanly with reepithelization within 8–10 days.
- It is superior to dithermy or freezing where tissue destruction is extensive and healing is more disturbed.
- Precise control over the area to be treated and depth of vapourisation.
- Squamocolumnar junction remains visible leaving the residual abnormality, if any, on the surface, which can be easily detected by cytology and colposcopy for subsequent redestruction.
- Cervical stenosis is not a problem.

Disadvantages
- May fail to eradicate the lesion completely, particularly if the lesion is very large.
- Potential danger to the operator.
- Inadvertent skin burns are known.
- Costly equipment.

4

Tubal
Infertility

Tubal pathology is a common factor in female infertility which may be the result of pelvic inflammatory disease, endometriosis and pelvic surgery causing pelvic adhesions or anatomical distortion of the fallopian tube and ovary. Such pelvic pathology may result in total or partial tubal occlusion, peritubal and periovarian adhesions or damage to ciliary and peristaltic functions of the tube. The consequences of such damage are infertility, ectopic pregnancy, pelvic pain and dyspareunia along with chronic ill health.

The approach to tubal infertility consists of
- Tubal patency tests for diagnostic evaluation
- Tubal reconstructive surgery for establishing patency.

TUBAL PATENCY TESTS
- To diagnose the tubal blocks in cases of infertility
- To confirm anatomical patency after reconstructive surgery on the fallopian tubes.

Methods
1. Hysterosalpingography
2. Sonosalpingography
3. Laparoscopic chromotubation
4. Saline test at laparotomy—transfundal/transcervical
5. Hysteroscopic cannulation of fallopian tubes
6. Salpingoscopy.

HYSTEROSALPINGOGRAPHY
It is radiological visualization of uterus and fallopian tubes after introducing radio-opaque dye through the cervix.

Time of procedure: Postmenstrual phase–between 4th and 7th day after the last day of the period.

If done in the premenstrual phase chances of:

a. Disturbing the conception

b. False positive results

Risk of endometriosis if done during bleeding phase.

Contraindications

- Vaginal bleeding
- Vaginal or cervical infection
- Genital tuberculosis
- Pelvic (adnexal) mass
- Pelvic infection
- Pregnancy (suspected)

Preparation

a. An enema or a strong purge to expel out gases from the colon to get a clear picture

b. Inj. Atropine to avoid cornual spasm.

Anaesthesia

No anaesthesia is required.

Instruments

- Instruments for visualizing cervix
- Tenaculum forceps
- Uterine sound
- Rubin's/Wilkinson's cannula
- Luer Lock syringe 20 ml and the radio-opaque dye

Steps

This procedure is done on the X-ray table.

1. Cervix is visualized.
2. Both the anterior and posterior lips of the cervix are caught by two tenaculum forceps.

3. Uterine sound is passed to assess the direction and the length of the uterus.
4. After confirming that the cannula can pass through the os, the syringe is filled with the dye.
5. The cannula is fitted to the syringe and all the air in the syringe and the cannula is completely expelled out. The cannula with the syringe attached is introduced through the cervix into the uterine cavity. The cork of the cannula should be adjusted to fit snugly on external os.
6. Slight pull is given on tenaculum forceps, while the cannula is gently pushed in, to avoid the leakage of the dye from the cervix in the vagina.
7. Under flouroscopic vision, the dye is slowly instilled into the uterus.
8. Radiological pictures are taken thereafter.

Interpretation

- Peritoneal spill on both sides indicates tubal patency.
- Any abnormality in the uterine cavity or the tubal lumen can be visualised.

Complications

Occasional patient may develop anaphylactic shock due to the sensitivity to the dye.

Advantages

- Simple, short procedure which does not require anaesthesia
- Exact location and the nature of the block can be known. Thus, further surgical treatment can be planned.
- Uterine abnormalities like bicornuate uterus, septate uterus, submucous fibroid, etc. can be diagnosed.
- Uterine synechiae can be diagnosed by honey-comb appearance.
- Unsuspected tubal tuberculosis can be diagnosed:
  - Rigid, lead-pipe appearance of the tube
  - Lymphatic extravasation of the dye
  - Tubal block

- Unsuspected genital tuberculosis can be diagnosed
  - Extravasation of the dye into the uterine wall
- Cervical incompetence can be diagnosed
  - Internal os wider than 8 mm (funnelling)
- Weak scar of previous caesarean section can be detected.
- May act therapeutically by breaking flimsy tubal adhesions.

Disadvantages
- False positive or false negative results are known.
- Cannot diagnose extra-tubal, extra-uterine pathologies, or pelvic adhesions.

LAPAROSCOPIC CHROMOTUBATION

This is comparatively a major procedure requiring hospitalization.

Time for surgery: It should be performed in the postmenstrual phase. However, it may be carried out premenstrually along with D and C.

Preoperative care and contraindications are discussed in details under laparoscopy operation.

Instruments

- Set of instruments for laparoscopy
- Set of instruments for hysterosalpingography.

Steps of Operation (For details *see* under laparoscopy)

1. Visualisation of pelvic organs through the telescope
2. Visualisation of cervix and introduction of Wilkinson's cannula into the uterine cavity vaginally.
3. Dilute methylene blue (few drops of methylene blue diluted in 20 ml of distilled water) is instilled into the uterine cavity. Care is taken to prevent the leakage of dye into the vagina.
4. The fallopian tubes are properly visualized through the telescope.
5. Spillage of the blue dye in the Pouch of Douglas through the fimbrial ends of the tubes is noted.

Advantages
- Along with the tubal patency, complete pelvic organs and the adnexa can be visualized.
- If the tubes are blocked, site and side of the block can be exactly located by noting bulging and bluish discolouration of tubes.
- Serosal surface of the tubes can be visualised.
- Any other pelvic pathology like pelvic adhesions, masses, genital tuberculosis, endometriosis, uterine malformations, ovarian pathology, etc. can be diagnosed.
- Certain therapeutic procedures like adhesiolysis, ovarian cysts puncture can be performed simultaneously. In short, it may prove as an alternative to the exploratory laparotomy in cases of infertility.
- Evidence of ovulation can directly be seen on the surface of ovary in the form of a corpus luteum.

Disadvantages
- Major procedure requiring general anaesthesia
- Risks more than with hysterosalpingography
- Hospitalisation for 24 hours required
- Experienced gynaecologist–endoscopist necessary
- Needs costly equipment

SONOSALPINGOGRAPHY (ASSESSMENT OF TUBAL PATENCY USING ULTRASOUND)
- Saline solution is instilled into the uterine cavity through a foley catheter.
- Transvaginal sonographic assessment is done.
- Air bubbles in periovarian space and fluid in pouch of Douglas indicate tubal patency.
- Turbulence in hydrosalpinx can be misdiagnosed as patent tube.
- This simple test is used as a screening method for evaluation of tubal factor.
- Good test for detection of intrauterine polyps.

SALINE TEST

This is a procedure to ascertain the tubal patency during laparotomy. This is not a primary method for diagnosing the tubal block, but it is a method of confirming and/or locating the tubal block during laparotomy performed for reconstructive surgery on tubes.

In this procedure, saline is injected through the fundus of the uterus during laparotomy and its spill or the distension of the tubes is noted to diagnose the patency or to locate the site of the blocks in the tubes (Table 4.1).

Indications

Suspected or diagnosed bilateral tubal blocks requiring reconstructive surgery on the tubes.

Instruments

- All instruments required for laparotomy
- Shirodkar's isthmus occluding clamp
- 18 G hypodermic needle, Leur Lock syringe 20 ml.
- Methylene blue solution in saline or distilled water.

Steps

1. Abdomen is opened
2. Uterus, tubes and ovaries are visualized and their external morphological appearances are noted.
3. With the help of Babcock's forceps, both the tubes are lifted and the fimbrial ends are rested on sponges.
4. Uterus is held by the Shirodkar's isthmus occluding clamp in such a way that the lower isthmic sleeves of the clamps hold the isthmus of the uterus firmly. Thus uterine contents do not leak out through the cervix. 18 G needle is introduced into the uterine cavity through the fundus of the uterus.
5. A syringe filled with dilute methylene blue solution is attached to the needle and the dye is injected into the uterine cavity.
6. Both the fallopian tubes are watched for the distension and spillage of dye from the fimbrial ends. The management is

Table 4.1: Saline test (interpretation and management)

	Observation	Inference	Treatment
a.	• No distension of tubes • Resistance during injection • Blanching of both cornual ends	Cornual block	• Implantation of tubes into uterus or • Tubocornual anastomosis
b.	• Tubes partially distended • No spillage	Midtubal block (isthmial or ampullary)	• Tubotubal anastomosis

c.	• Distension of whole tube
	• No spillage
		Fimbrial block	• Salpingostomy
			  Cuff
			  Linear

d.	• Spillage seen	One or both tubes patent	• No treatment • Salpingolysis if adhesions

e.	• No distension of tubes
	• No resistance during injection
	• No spillage
		Clamp loosely or wrongly applied
		Vaginal leakage
			• Proper application of clamp
			  and retesting the tubal
			  patency

planned according to the interpretation of the test (Table 4.1).

Alternatively, Foley's catheter can be introduced transcervically. Bulb of the catheter is inflated to block the internal os of the cervix. Then methylene blue solution is instilled into the uterine cavity for testing tubal patency.

Therapeutic Benefits of Diagnostic Tests

About 1/3rd patients conceive after tubal patency tests. Possibilities for such beneficial effect are:

- Separation of the mild agglutinations of the tubal folds.
- Displacement of the inspissated mucous from narrower to wider portions, and thus opening fimbrial adhesions.
- Opening of flimsy intraluminal adhesions in the tube.

TUBAL RECONSTRUCTIVE SURGERY

The surgery of choice in tubal reconstructive surgery depends upon the site of tubal occlusion.

Procedures

1. Salpingolysis and ovariolysis
2. Fimbrioplasty
3. Salpingoneostomy (salpingostomy)
4. Tubal anastomosis
5. Tubouterine implantation.

Selection of Patients

1. *Age:* Patient should be under 40 years of age.
2. *General health:* Patient's fitness is assessed for:
    - Surgery
    - Subsequent pregnancy
3. Other factors like anovulation, male factor, etc. responsible for infertility must be ruled out.
4. *Tubal assessment by:*
    - Laparoscopy

Good prognosis is indicated by:
- Healthy fimbria
- Length of tube >4 cm
- Absence of peritubal adhesions
- Absence of tuberculosis

Advantage of laparoscopy
- *Patent tubes:* Surgery is avoided
- Grossly damaged tubes: Laparotomy avoided
- Hysterosalpingography: For the information about interstitial portion of the tube and tubal lining.

Timing of Surgery

Ideally, the surgery is performed during the proliferative phase of the cycle. Vascularity being less during this phase, technically there are less problems and the chances of postoperative adhesions formation are avoided. Also, due to oestrogenic influence, healing is better. Oestrogen helps ciliogenesis also.

Principles of Microsurgery

1. Adequate surgical exposure
   - Elevation of the uterus to a constant operating plane by vaginal packing or pelvic packing.
   - A generous low transverse incision
   - Use of four bladed retractor
2. Prevention of peritoneal surface damage
   - Gentle tissue handling
   - Use of delicate instruments
   - Continuous irrigation
3. Continuous irrigation of pelvic structures is done with isotonic solutions by a cannula connected to a intravenous infusion set. Heparin 5000 IU added to Ringer lactate solution is used for this purpose.
4. Use of non tissue reactive fine suture material (6/0 or 8/0) on fine needles.
5. *Meticulous haemostasis:* Use of microelectrode for cutting and coagulation.

6. *Optical magnification:* This allows better definition of tissue layers and greater accuracy of tissue alignment.
   - Operating microscope
   - Magnification loupe
7. Closure of all peritoneal surfaces to prevent adhesions
8. Correct opposition of tubal ends
9. Use of adjuvants
   - To prevent pelvic adhesions:
     - Corticosteroids–systemic or peritoneal
     - Dextran solution (32%)
   - *Polythelene intratubal stent:* Stents are used only intraoperatively except in cornual implantation.
10. *Postoperative:*
    - Postoperative hydrotubation is generally not performed to minimize the chances of infection.
    - Prophylactic antibiotics
    - Prophylactic steroids
11. *Follow-up:* Assessment of tubal patency by laparoscopy/ hysterosalpingography after a period of 6 months.

SALPINGOLYSIS AND OVARIOLYSIS

This comprises of division of adhesions surrounding the tube or ovary. It can be performed during laparotomy or laparoscopy.

The adhesions are lifted away from surrounding tissues with the help of glass rod and are divided with microelectrodes and cutting diathermy. Careful reperitonization of all raw surfaces is done in the end. The success depends upon the severity of the adhesions.

FIMBRIOPLASTY

- This procedure is performed where fimbrial end though patent is constricted due to adherent fimbria by a firm scar.
- The avascular line of agglutination can be seen under magnification and severed with the microelectrode.
- Partial enfolding of fimbria resulting in a constricting ring compressing a tuft of fimbria requires incision of such ring after which normal looking fimbria pop out.

SALPINGOSTOMY

It is performed for totally occluded distal tube. The lines of fimbrial agglutination, which meet at central point, are identified well under magnification.

Outer end of the tube is visualised microscopically and incisions are made along the scar lines with microelectrodes. The fimbria are dissected free and everted. Sometimes suturing is required to maintain this eversion of fimbria.

TUBAL ANASTOMOSIS

- Uteroisthmic
- Uteroampullary
- Isthmo-isthmic
- Ampullo-isthmic
- Ampullo-ampullary

Consists of

- Accurate excision of blocked tissue
- Precise opposition of the segments
- Careful suturing through myosalpinx, excluding endosalpinx
- Suturing the serosal layer

This surgery is commonly indicated for reversal of tubectomy.

Best results are obtained where minimal destruction of the isthmial portion has taken place. Damage is minimal with the clip sterilization (0.4 mm). Tubal damage by Fallop rings and Pomeroy's technique is almost the same (3 cm). Cauterization damages much larger segment of the tube.

Mostly performed through laparotomy. Laparoscopic microsurgical tubal reanastomosis also gives good results in skilled hands.

TUBAL IMPLANTATION

This is performed for cornual block. There are two techniques:
- Cornual implantation
- Posterior fundal implantation.

CORNUAL IMPLANTATION

- Creation of a stoma in the cornu by sharp excision or by using reamer.
- *Implantation of isthmus or ampulla:* Ampullary implantation is easier due to its wider diameter.
- The end of the resected tube is longitudinally split to make a fish mouth. A suture is placed through each split flap. A polythelene splint is placed through both the tubes making a ring in the uterine cavity for its subsequent removal after 4 months hysteroscopically.
- The flaps are implanted through the stoma into the uterine cavity by bringing out the sutures through anterior and posterior uterine walls respectively.

Disadvantages
- More bleeding during procedure
- Low success rate
- Subsequent delivery by caesarean section.

POSTERIOR FUNDAL IMPLANTATION

- Instead of creating a stoma in the uterine wall, a posterior transverse fundal incision is taken.
- Ampullary portion is implanted.
- Myometrium between the implanted fallopian tubes is sutured in two layers.

5

Gynaecological Endoscopy

Endoscopies are procedures in which internal organs are visualized through telescope. Most operative procedures are currently being performed endoscopically.

LAPAROSCOPY

Indications

Diagnostic

- *Pelvic pain:*
  - *Acute:* To differentiate acute pelvic infection from chronic leaking ectopic pregnancy.
  - *Chronic:* To diagnose PID, adhesions, endometriosis, pelvic congestion syndrome, etc.
- Unruptured ectopic gestation
- Genital tuberculosis
- *Adnexal masses:* Tubo-ovarian masses, ovarian endometrioma, ovarian neoplasm.

Evaluation

- *Infertility:* Tubal patency, peritubal adhesions, tubo-ovarian mass, pelvic tuberculosis, endometriosis, polycystic ovaries
- *Amenorrhoea:* Mullerian agenesis, dysgenetic gonads, genital tuberculosis
- Congenital malformations of genital tract
- Uterine perforation following surgical MTP
  - Extent of damage
  - Amount of bleeding

Therapeutic (Operative laparoscopy)

- *Tubal:*
  - Sterilization by applying rings, clips,
  - Ectopic pregnancy
  - Tubal reconstructive surgery, adhesiolysis
- *Endometriosis:* Fulguration of patches, endometrioma
- *Ovaries:*
  - Follicular puncture with microcauterization in cases of polycystic ovaries
  - Aspiration of small ovarian cysts, ovarian cystectomy, oophorectomy
- Removal of misplaced IUCD from peritoneal cavity
- *Biopsies:* Ovaries, pelvic peritoneum, etc.
- *Uterine surgery:* Myomectomy, hysterectomy
- Pelvic floor repair, retropubic cystourethropexy for stress urinary incontinence
- Uterosacral transsection for dysmenorrhoea
- Uterine suspension.

Contraindications

All the contraindications are relative and the list given may change according to the experience of the laparoscopist and the anaesthetist.

- Cardiorespiratory diseases
- Palpable abdominal masses
- Advanced malignancies
- Tubercular peritonitis
- Umbilical/hiatus hernia
- Previous abdominal surgery
- Gross obesity

Anaesthesia

Usually performed under general anaesthesia. Sterilisation can be performed under local anaesthesia.

Time for Procedure

When it is to be combined with the endometrial biopsy for the investigations of infertility, it is to be performed in the postovulatory phase. Sterilization is to be performed in the post menstrual period to avoid the chance of operating in the early pregnancy.

Procedure

1. Instruments: Laparoscopy instruments (Fig. 5.1).
2. Curved incision at the lower border of umbilicus.
3. Insertion of Veress needle while lifting the abdominal wall. Test with saline drop to confirm intraperitoneal entry.
4. Creation of pneumoperitoneum slowly by using CO_2, assure uniform distension of abdomen and obliteration of liver dullness.

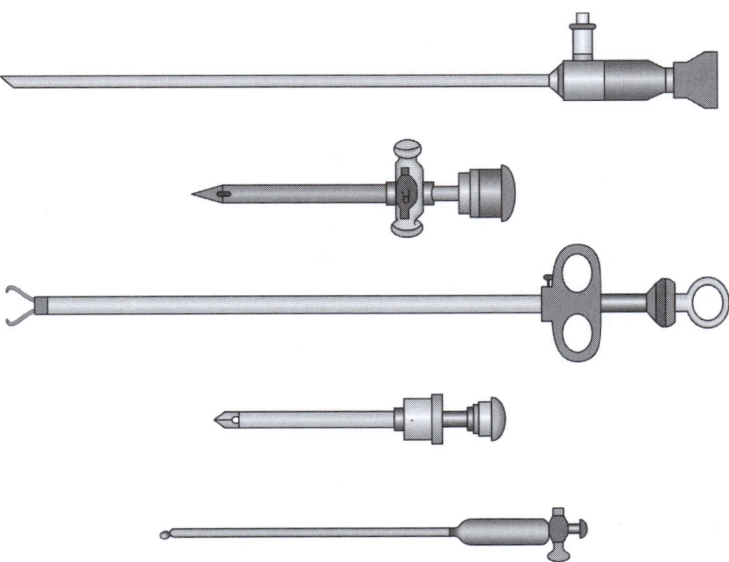

Fig. 5.1: Laparoscopy instruments. 1. Laparoscope; 2. Trocar and cannula 3. Ring applicator; 4. Second puncture trocar and cannula; 5. Veress needle

5. Trocar insertion while lifting the abdominal wall
   - Extended index finger used as a guide and palm supports the trocar
   - 45° inclination towards pelvis
6. Introduction of telescope, with fiberoptic cable connected to light source
7. Visualization of pelvic organs using uterine manipulator and performing operative procedures through additional ports.
8. The gas from the peritoneal cavity should be expelled out completely, lest prolonged shoulder pain and abdominal discomfort should persist. After completion of the procedure, the patient should be brought to horizontal position and telescope in the cannula should be replaced by trocar, which opens its valve and lets the gas out through its hollow canal.

Complications

Operative

- Subcutaneous introduction of gas–mediastinal emphysema
- Uterine perforation by manipulator
- Bowel, stomach, omental sac, urinary bladder injury
- Gas embolism
- Injury to parietal or visceral blood vessels causing intraperitoneal or extraperitoneal haemorrhage
- Accidental puncture of inferior vena cava or aorta
- Burns to the viscera by cautery; commoner with unipolar cautery
- Cardiopulmonary accidents
- Omental prolapse

Postoperative

- Infection
- Secondary intraperitoneal haemorrhage
- Intestinal or omental adhesions at umbilicus

Side Effects

Shoulder pain for few days due to residual gas settling under and irritating diaphragm.

VIDEO ENDOSCOPY

Endoscopic surgery is being done with endovision video camera, which is attached to the eye piece of the telescope. The endoscopic picture seen on monitor guides the operating team for performing various operative procedures.

Advantages
- Minimally invasive surgery
- Postural comforts to the surgeon
- Good teaching tool
- Videographic documentation possible.

LAVH (LAPAROSCOPIC ASSISTED VAGINAL HYSTERECTOMY)

Vaginal hysterectomy is associated with less postoperative morbidity as compared to the abdominal one. However, it is difficult and risky in the presence of adhesions and when removal of adnexa is necessary as in endometriosis. LAVH is helpful in these situations.

Aims

To convert
- Abdominal hysterectomy into a vaginal procedure
- Difficult vaginal hysterectomy into an easy one.

Laparoscopic Hysterectomy

Uterine arteries divided laparoscopically

LAVH

Uterine vessels secured vaginally

Advantages
- Large incision avoided
- Less bleeding
- Less postoperative pain
- Rapid recovery
- Shorter hospital stay
- Less adhesion formation

- Less chances of infection
- Cosmetic

Disadvantage
- Skilled surgeons required, sophisticated equipment and instruments required, operating time prolonged, cost more.

Principles

1. Insertion of 10 mm laparoscope with attached video camera
2. Suprapubic insertion of 5 mm trocar for suction irrigation
3. Insertion of lateral trocars on either side under vision avoiding the inferior epigastric vessels
4. Upper pedicles are divided after securing them with staples, electrodiathermy or endosutures
5. Uterovesical pouch is opened.
6. Uterus is delivered vaginally after dividing the lower pedicles.

HYSTEROSCOPY

This is a procedure for endoscopic visualisation of uterine cavity and endocervix.

Indications

Diagnostic

1. To diagnose intrauterine pathologies like polyps, submucous fibromyoma, carcinoma
2. To obtain biopsy from suspected area
3. Infertility evaluation–in combination with laparoscopy
4. Diagnosis and treatment of intrauterine synaechae
5. Menstrual abnormalities–dysfunctional uterine bleeding, intermenstrual bleeding
6. Abnormal uterine/vaginal bleeding
7. Recurrent abortions–to exclude septum or submucous fibroid
8. Puerperal bleeding–to rule out retained products of conception or any other intrauterine lesion.

Therapeutic Surgical

1. Subseptate uterus–excision of septum
2. Detection and recovery of misplaced intrauterine contraceptive device
3. Adhesiolysis in Aschermann's syndrome.
4. Resection of submucous myoma
5. Transcervical resection of endometrium (TCRE) for menorrhagia
6. Laser ablation of endometrium
7. Tubal cannulation for medial tubal block.

Contraindications

1. Pregnancy
2. Infection
3. Heavy uterine bleeding–presence of blood in large amount may obliterate the view
4. History of recurrent perforations.

Timing of Procedure

It may be performed at any time depending upon indication. However, postmenstrual phase is ideal as tubal ostei are readily identified.

Anaesthesia

Local anaesthesia–paracervical block

Instruments

- Telescope–4 mm diameter with sheath 5–6 mm diameter
- Fibreoptic light transmission system
- Distending medium–vide infra
- Operating channel
- Operating instruments–resectoscope, cautery electrode
- 150 W light source
- Portioadaptors cervix
- Sim's speculum, volsellum, set of dilators, uterine sound.

Gaseous Distension

Hysteroflator is used for distending uterine cavity by CO_2. Flow should not exceed 100 ml/min. and should be under low pressure. High pressure and rapid flow are dangerous and may lead to hypercarbia.

Fluid Distension

- Glycine
- High molecular weight dextran 30% (Hyskon)
- Dextrose 5% in water

Steps of Operation

1. Cervix is visualized and anterior lip of cervix is held with volsellum.
2. Paracervical block is given.
3. Sounding of the uterine cavity is done.
4. Cervix is dilated as required.
5. If cervix is patulous (where dilatation is not required), it is sealed by cervical suction cup.
6. Telescope is introduced into uterine cavity.
7. Uterine cavity is distended.
8. Visualization of uterine cavity is done. Tubal ostei are seen. Uterine septum, polyps, adhesions, submucus myoma are detected
9. Necessary surgical procedures are carried out.

Complications

a. Perforation of the uterus
b. Infection
c. Complications due to distending medium—CO_2 flow at high rate under high pressure is dangerous. It may lead to acidosis and cardiac arrhythmias due to hypercarbia.
d. Fluid overload due to fluid distending media.

6 | Hysterectomy

Hysterectomy is an operation to remove the uterus.

Types

1. *Total hysterectomy:* Uterine body and the cervix are removed.
2. *Subtotal hysterectomy:* Only uterine body is removed, while cervix is retained. Although this is technically easy to perform, it is not performed, as later on if the stump of the cervix develops malignancy, it becomes very difficult to treat it surgically as well as radiotherapeutically, due to its altered anatomic relations.
3. *Panhysterectomy:* Uterus, cervix, both fallopian tubes and ovaries are removed. (Total hysterectomy with bilateral salpingo-oophorectomy).
4. *Radical hysterectomy:* Uterus, cervix, both tubes and ovaries, upper 2/3 of vagina, parametrium and the pelvic lymph nodes are removed. It is performed for selected cases of malignancy of cervix and endometrium.

Routes
   i. Abdominal
   ii. Vaginal
   iii. Laparoscopic

Indications
1. Non-neoplastic Conditions
   a. *Dysfunctional uterine bleeding:* Functional menorrhagia in perimenopausal woman uncontrolled by medical management leading to significant anaemia.

53

b. Adenomyosis causing intractable menorrhagia.

c. Episodes of postmenopausal bleeding in absence of detectable pathology.

d. Genital prolapse in an elderly and parous woman.

2. Inflammatory Diseases

a. Pelvic inflammatory diseases failing to resolve or recurring frequently after adequate medical treatment and persistent tubo-ovarian masses producing distressing symptoms which are unrelieved by conservative management.

b. *Pyometra:* Specially in an old woman where no apparent cause has been detected and infection has been brought under control.

c. Some cases of genital tuberculosis with persistent pelvic masses after chemotherapy.

3. Benign Neoplastic Conditions

a. *Uterine fibromyoma:* Symptomatic fibromyoma, age 40+ years, family completed.

b. Benign ovarian neoplasm in perimenopausal woman.

4. Premalignant Conditions

a. *CIN III of uterine cervix:* Elderly and parous woman, with associated gynecological conditions, recurrent disease after excision.

b. Adenocarcinoma in situ of cervix.

c. Endometrial hyperplasia with atypia.

5. Malignant Diseases

a. Carcinoma cervix

b. Carcinoma endometrium

c. Choriocarcinoma

d. Other uterine malignancies

e. Malignant ovarian tumours.

6. *Prophylactic*

Vesicular mole in an elderly (age 40 + years regardless of parity) and parous woman (parity 3 + regardless of age)–to minimise the risk of choriocarcinoma.

7. *Traumatic*

  a. *Obstertric injuries:* Rupture of the uterus associated with uncontrollable haemorrhage or haematoma due to the torn uterine vessel. Usually these rents can be repaired, but if bleeding is uncontrolled, hysterectomy is performed as an emergency life saving procedure.

  b. *Operative injuries:* Rarely perforation of the uterus during D and C may call for hysterectomy; particularly if a myoma or a submucous fibroid gets injured.

  c. *Accidental injuries:* The main indication is rupture or severe damage to the uterine vessels.

8. *Congenital Defects*

  a. Atresia of the cervix or lower genital tract leading to the damage to the uterus after haematometra.

  b. Rudimentory horn of the uterus causing haematometra or ectopic pregnancy.

9. *Obstetric Conditions*

Vide obstetric hysterectomy.

Time of Surgery

Postmenstrual phase is preferred; as there is less congestion and hence less operative oozing.

Preoperative Preparations

  1. Patient's haemogram and urine examination should be done and any pathology should be corrected.
  2. General fitness of the patient should be ascertained for anaesthesia and to withstand the major surgery.
  3. Grouping and cross-matching of the blood.

4. *Diet:* Previous night patient is given a light diet, after which she is kept nil by mouth.
5. Sedative/tranquilizer is given previous night.
6. *Bowels:* Mostly, preoperative simple enema is considered sufficient. However, in radical surgery, previous night purge following morning bowel wash is required.
7. A good hot water bath is given prior to the surgery.
8. *Preparation of the parts:* Cleaning of the skin over operative field by antiseptic lotions.
9. *Bladder:* It is preferred to catheterize the bladder on table and retain the catheter during surgery in cases of abdominal approach. This helps to keep the bladder empty throughout the operation; minimizing the risk of bladder injury. Also assessment of extent of perfusion can be made by noting the urine output.
10. *Premedication:*
   a. Inj. Atropine 0.6 mg is given intramuscularly about 20 minutes prior to surgery.
   b. Inj. Pethidine 50 mg, Inj. Diazepam 10 mg or Inj. Pentazocain 30 mg.
11. A written informed consent for the operation.

Anaesthesia

General, spinal or epidural anaesthesia.

ABDOMINAL HYSTERECTOMY

Instruments

- Sponge holders
- BP handle no. 4
- Scalpel blade no. 22
- Dissecting forceps–toothed and plain
- Artery forceps–straight and curved
- Kocher's clamps–straight and curved
- Allis forceps
- Needle holders
- Mayo's trocar pointed half circle needles

- Curved cutting needles
- Curved round body needles
- Bladder retractor–large and small
- Self retaining abdominal retractor
- Right angle retractors.

Steps of Operation

A. *Opening the Abdomen*

B. *Removal of Uterus*

1. After opening the abdomen, the parietes are retracted by self-retaining retractor and bladder is retracted with bladder retractor.
2. Uterus, tubes, ovaries and other pelvic organs are inspected.
3. Pedicles are clamped, cut between the Kocher's forceps and ligated.
   The different pedicles divided and ligated are as follows:
   Pedicle I → Round ligament.
   Pedicle II → Ovarian ligament and Fallopian tubes if ovaries are to be retained as in total hysterectomy.
   Infundibulopelvic ligaments if ovaries are to be removed
4. Uterovesical pouch of peritoneum is opened and the urinary bladder is pushed below the level of the cervix.
5. Remaining two pedicles are cut between the clamps and ligated.
   Pedicle III → Uterine vessels
   Pedicle IV → Uterosacral and Mackenrodt's ligaments
6. Vagina is opened below the level of the cervix between two Allis forceps, cut transversely and the uterus is removed.

C. *Closure of Vaginal Vault*

1. The last pedicle is secured to the angle of the vagina.
2. Vagina is closed.
3. Pelvic peritoneum may be closed, keeping all the stumps of pedicles extraperitoneal.

D. *Closure of Abdomen*

Postoperative Care

1. Patient is kept nil by mouth in the immediate postoperative period and the nutrition and hydration is maintained by parenteral fluid therapy.
2. For first 24 hours, the patient is advised to take complete bed rest; but from the second day onwards, early ambulation is encouraged.
3. On first day, sometimes patient is unable to pass urine, mostly because she is not used to pass urine in recumbent position. Simpler methods like little propped up position, sounds of running water, etc. should be tried before catheterizing the bladder.
4. After the peristaltic movements are established, the patient is given oral feeds. They are started from sips of water and gradually changed over to the full diet.
5. Suitable antibiotic is given prophylactically.
6. After 8 days, the stitches are removed.

Complications

Immediate

1. Intraoperative haemorrhage
2. Haematoma formation–subcutaneous and under the rectus sheath.
3. *Infection*
   a. Wound infection
   b. Pelvic infection
   c. Peritonitis
   d. Urinary tract infection
4. *Abdominal distention*
   a. Peritonitis
   b. Intestinal obstruction
   c. Paralytic ileus
5. Thrombophlebitis

Delayed

1. Chronic abdominal pain due to adhesions
2. Incisional hernia
3. Vault prolapse–if enterocele is overlooked.

WERTHEIM'S RADICAL HYSTERECTOMY

This is abdominal radical hysterectomy done for carcinoma of the cervix, mostly for stages Ib and IIa; and carcinoma of endometrium stage II.

Preoperative

a. Intravenous pyelography is performed to locate the ureters and to exclude obstructive uropathy.
b. Bowels are emptied by Bowel wash followed by overnight purge.
c. On the table, vagina may be packed tightly under anaesthesia to lift up the uterus and to enable removal of the greater portion of the vagina.
d. Foley's self retaining catheter is introduced into the bladder.

Principles of Surgical Procedure

1. *Operability is Assessed*

   a. Palpation of liver, spleen, kidneys, diaphragm and pelvic and para-aortic nodes
   b. Assessing mobility of uterus and cervix.
   c. Opening the uterovesical pouch and separating urinary bladder from the cervix.

2. *Wide Resection of Tissues Comprising*

   a. Uterus with cervix, both tubes, ovaries and upper 2/3rds of vagina
   b. As much parametrial tissue as possible
   c. *Lymph nodes:* Obturator, external iliac, internal iliac

   This is achieved by clamping the pedicles as laterally as possible, dividing uterine artery at its origin, dissecting the ureter by opening the ureteric canal to its entry into the bladder and extensive dissection of the vagina by separating urinary bladder anteriorly and the rectum posteriorly.

To prevent the spillage of the malignant cells, Berkeley Bonney Wertheim's hysterectomy clamp or Myxter's forceps is applied to the vagina, below which vagina is opened and cut.

As far as possible, specimen is removed en bloc to avoid spillage of malignant cells.

Postoperative Care
- Adequate replacement of blood
- Continuous drainage of bladder by Foley's catheter for 7 to 10 days.

Complications
1. Primary mortality high
2. Primary haemorhage
3. Injury to rectum, urinary bladder and ureters
4. *Ureteric fistulae:*
    a. Direct injury–cutting, crushing or ligation of ureter.
    b. Indirect injury–avascular necrosis due to stripping off the ureter completely of its blood supply.

Further Management
Postoperative radiotherapy is given if lymph nodes show malignant infiltration.

VAGINAL HYSTERECTOMY
Indications
- Usually vaginal hysterectomy is performed in cases of genital prolapse.
- In selected cases with no cervical descent, this route may be preferred for other indications like DUB also.

Time for Surgery
Preferably postmenstrual.

This route was avoided earlier in cases of

- Large uterus
- Uterine tumours
- Ovarian tumours
- Previous abdominal surgery resulting in fixity of uterus due to adhesions
- Malignancies
- Nulliparous patient with no cervical descent.

Currently, with the help of laparoscope this route can be used for these cases also.

Preoperative

- Cases with decubitus ulcers in the vagina are to be deferred till the ulcers heal completely.
- Antiseptic vaginal packing overnight.

Anaesthesia

General or spinal anaesthesia.

Instruments

In addition to general instruments:

- Sim's/Auvard's speculum
- Volsellum
- Right angle retractor
- Jayle's vaginal self-retaining retractor
- Metal catheter
- Bladder sound

Steps of Operation

1. Patient's legs are tied in lithotomy position after she is given suitable anaesthesia.
2. Urinary bladder is catheterized.
3. Sim's/Auvard's speculum is inserted into the vagina, cervix is held by volsellum and bladder extent is ascertained by bladder sound.
4. Anterior vaginal wall is incised transversely below the bladder sulcus on the cervix.

5. Incision is extended posteriorly in a circular fashion.
6. Vagina is separated posteriorly, Pouch of Douglas is identified and opened.
7. Anteriorly, vesicocervical ligament is incised and urinary bladder is pushed high up.
8. Vesicouterine pouch of peritoneum is identified and opened.
9. Urinary bladder is retracted behind the right angle retractor.
10. Uterosacral and Mackenrodt's ligaments are clamped, divided and transfixed on both sides.
11. Uterine vessels are clamped, cut and transfixed on both sides.
12. Upper part of broad ligament including round ligament and fallopian tube is clamped, cut and transfixed when ovaries are retained. Infundibulopelvic ligaments are clamped, cut and transfixed when ovaries are removed.
13. Peritoneum may be sutured and the pedicles are extraperitonized.
14. All pedicles from either side are brought together in the midline.
15. Vaginal edges are approximated.
16. Tight pack may be kept in the vagina for 6–12 hours.

Complications

Intraoperative

a. Haemorrhage
b. Injury to the urinary bladder
c. Injury to rectum
d. Anaesthetic complications

Postoperative

a. Retention of urine
b. Urinary infection
c. Pelvic infection/abscess
d. Secondary haemorrhage due to infection.

Delayed

a. Vault prolapse

b. Vault granulation

Table 6.1 shows the comparison of two rules of hysterectomy.

Table 6.1: Abdominal vs vaginal hysterectomy	
Abdominal	*Vaginal*
1. Large uterus with tumours can be removed	1. Uterus should be normal sized or just enlarged
2. Adhesions of the uterus can be released	2. Uterus must be mobile and free of adhesions; hence not suitable in cases of previous abdominal surgery
3. Suitable for: • Fibroids • Ovarian tumours • Malignancies • Pelvic inflammatory disease	3. Suitable for: • Prolapse • Dysfunctional uterine bleeding
4. Vaginal wall prolapse cannot be repaired satisfactorily	4. Vaginal wall prolapse can be repaired properly
5. Radical surgery easier	5. Radical surgery difficult
6. Complications like unexpected bleeding can be tackled easily	6. Difficult to control unexpected haemorrhage. Laparotomy may be required.
7. Difficult in obese women	7. Preferred in obese women
8. Postoperatively patient more uncomfortable due to more handling of the bowels and due to the abdominal incision	8. Convalescence smooth with rapid recovery (due to less handling of the bowels). Minimal pain as no abdominal wound
9. Complications due to abdominal scar like wound dehiscence, incisional hernia are known	9. No scar complications; except secondary haemorrhage from infected vaginal incision
10. Patient worried about abdominal stitches and scar	10. 'Stitchless' operation for patient, scar not visible

Laparoscopic hysterectomy and laparoscopically assisted vaginal hysterectomy (LAVH) are new techniques for hysterectomy with very small incision, shorter hospital stay and less postoperative morbidity.

Specially trained skilled surgical team and costly equipment are required.

Complications can be more in poorly selected cases and surgery performed by less skilled persons (vide details on page 49 and 50).

7

Genital Prolapse

There is a wide range of operations for repairing genital prolapsed from which a proper surgical procedure is selected for an individual case. The selection of the operative procedure depends upon the following factors:

1. Age
2. Parity
3. *Type of prolapse:*
   - Uterine descent
   - Cystocoele
   - Rectocoele
   - Enterocoele
   - Vault prolapse
4. Extent of cervical elongation
5. Associated pathology
   - Menstrual disorders
   - Cervical pathology
   - New growths

Selection of Treatment Modality

1. *Young patients desiring further pregnancies:* Prolapse repair with conservation of the uterus is preferred. It can be performed by two routes:
   - *Vaginal route:*
     - Fothergill's (Manchester) operation
     - Shirodkar's modification of Fothergill's operation
   - *Abdominal route:*
     - Shirodkar's posterior sling
     - Purandare's cervicopexy
     - Khanna's sling

2. Elderly patient having completed her family:
   - Mayo-Ward's operation
3. Old frail patients unfit for major surgery and where sexual activity is of no concern
   - Le Fort's operation
4. Patients unfit or unwilling for any surgery
   - Ring pessary
5. Genital prolapse associated with pregnancy and puerperium
   - Ring pessary

MAYO-WARD'S OPERATION

This is a vaginal operation performed for genital prolapse; which includes:

   i. Vaginal hysterectomy
   ii. Anterior colporrhaphy
   iii. Posterior colpoperineorrhaphy

Selection of Patients

- Age 35 years or more
- Completed the family
- Associated symptoms like distressing menorrhagia or leucorrhoea due to unhealthy cervix.

Steps of Operations

1. *Vaginal Hysterectomy*

After removal of the uterus, the pedicles on either side are tied to each other in the midline.

2. *Anterior Colporrhaphy*

Done for cystocoele repair

- The extent of the cystocoele is noted by means of bladder sound.
- Inverted 'T' shaped incision is taken on the anterior vaginal wall.
- Vesicocervical ligament is cut.

- The urinary bladder is dissected and pushed up.
- Buttressing sutures are taken for the pubocervical fascia.
- Redundant vaginal wall is excised and the vagina is closed.

3. *Posterior Colpoperineorrhaphy*

For rectocoele/enterocoele repair

- Transverse incision is taken on the mucocutaneous junction of the posterior vaginal wall at the level of myritiformis carunculae and the perineal skin.
- The incision is extended in the vagina in a triangular fashion on the posterior vaginal wall, the highest point of which should be above the posterior wall laxity.
- Rectum is separated from the posterior vaginal wall.
- Bellies of the levator ani muscles are identified to bring them together in the midline by interrupted sutures between vagina and rectum.
- Redundant posterior vaginal wall is excised.
- Vaginal edges are sutured in longitudinal fashion.
- Suturing of the perineal muscles and skin edges is done in layers.

Postoperative

1. Tight vaginal pack for 24 hours to prevent haemorrhage in the vesicovaginal or rectovaginal spaces.
2. Self-retaining catheter in the bladder with continuous drainage for 48–72 hours.
3. Removal of perineal stitches after 5 to 7 days.

FOTHERGILL'S (MANCHESTER) OPERATION
Selection of Patients

- Young patient
- There is elongation of cervix
- Patient is desirous of conserving the uterus
- No other uterine pathology demanding removal of uterus
- Significant vaginal wall prolapse.

Principles of Operation

- Cervical dilatation
- Cervical amputation
- Covering the raw cervix with vaginal flaps
- Shortening and advancement of Mackenrodt's ligament in front of the cervix, which maintains the anteversion of the uterus
- Anterior colporrhaphy
- Posterior colpoperineorrhaphy.

Complications

Immediate

- Haemorrhage
- Injury to the bladder or rectum
- Infection

Delayed

- Recurrence of prolapse
- During subsequent pregnancy:
  - Cervical incompetence resulting due to high amputation of cervix can lead to midtrimester abortions or preterm deliveries.
  - Cervical dystocia due to the fibrosis of cervix
- Infertility due to cervical factor.

SHIRODKAR'S MODIFICATION OF FOTHERGILL'S OPERATION

Selection of Patient

- Young patient
- Minimum cervical elongation
- Significant vaginal wall prolapse.

Modifications

- Cervical amputation is not done.
- Shortening and advancement of uterosacral ligaments is done anterior to the cervix.

Advantage
Complications of cervical amputation are avoided.

SHIRODKAR'S POSTERIOR SLING
Selection of Patient
- Young patient desiring further pregnancy
- Not much cervical elongation
- Minimal vaginal wall prolapse.

Principles of Operation
- Abdominal procedure for suspending uterus and cervix with a mersilene sling
- The sling is fixed to the posteror surface of isthmus anteriorly and to the anterior longitudinal ligament on the sacral promontary posteriorly, reinforcing the uterosacral ligaments.
- On left side, due to the presence of the pelvic portion of the descending colon, the sling has to pass through a loop created by mersilene tape on the psoas muscle.
- Shirodkar's ligature carriers are required for this operation.

The patients who have undergone this type of repair can undergo vaginal deliveries in subsequent pregnancies.

Disadvantages
- Major abdominal procedure
- Sling material costly
- Unsuitable for associated vaginal wall prolapse of considerable degree.

Complications
- Injury to genitofemoral nerve, external iliac vessels or ureter
- Retroperitoneal haematoma

To reduce the complexity and complications of the procedure on left side, currently only unilateral right sided posterior sling is being practiced.

PURANDARE'S CERVICOPEXY

Selection of Cases

- Young patient desiring further pregnancy
- Cervical elongation minimal
- Minimal vaginal wall prolapse

Principles of Surgery

- Transverse abdominal incision is taken for the skin and rectus sheath.
- Strips in the aponeurosis of the external oblique muscle about 1 cm width are prepared on both sides and held with stay sutures.
- Long curved artery forceps are passed through internal inguinal ring extraperitoneally and the sling is brought through broad ligament to the anterior surface of the isthmus.
- Sling is anchored to the anterior surface of the isthmus.

Advantages

- Natural fascial strips
- Technically easy
- With rise in intra-abdominal pressure, instead of pushing the uterus down, the sling pulls the cervix up due to contraction of the rectus muscle.

Disadvantages

- Incidence of recurrence is high.
- Associated vaginal wall prolapse cannot be corrected.
- Unsuitable for asthenic patient as fascial strips also are asthenic. This problem can be overcome by using mersilene tape.

MOSCHCOWITZ OPERATION

This is an abdominal operation for the repair of enterocoele.

Indications

- This operation is performed when enterocoele is associated with other pelvic conditions requiring laparotomy or abdominal hysterectomy.

- Unsuspected enterocoele diagnosed during abdominal surgery.

Principles of Operation

1. *Position:* Trendelenburg position
2. If uterus is retained, it is held up and forward; if it is removed, then posterior wall of the vaginal vault is held by Allis forceps.
3. A purse-string suture is placed by no. 0 silk to encircle the Pouch of Douglas. The suture is started at the bottom of the sac. These sutures should include only peritoneum laterally so as to avoid injury to the ureters; and only serosa over the rectum.
4. Successive purse-string sutures are placed till the region of the uterosacral ligaments is reached. Good firm bites are taken through the ligaments and into the posterior surface of vagina. The last; highest suture should be tied without tension.

LE FORT'S OPERATION (COLPOCLEISIS)
Principles

Denuding areas of anterior and posterior vaginal walls and approximating them; thus obliterating the vaginal canal, leaving two narrow lateral tunnels for drainage.

Preoperative evaluation of cervix and uterus by cytology, USG and curettage if required should be performed to exclude occult malignancy.

Suitable only for very old patients medically unfit for surgery, with complete prolapse and who have completed their sexual life.

Advantages
- Quick procedure
- Can be performed under local anaesthesia.

Disadvantages
- Obliteration of vaginal canal terminates sexual life.
- Incidence of stress incontinence is high.

Pessary for Correction of Genital Prolapse

Rubber ring pessary is used for this purpose. When introduced in vagina, it stretches the vagina and rests on the levator ani muscles to prevent the prolapse. It is sterilized by chemical methods, i.e. immersing in antiseptic solution for 30 minutes.

Uses

- *Pregnancy:* Until uterus becomes abdominal
- Puerperium
- When surgery has to be deferred.

Selection of Size

The distance between the posterior fornix and the lower end of pubic symphysis is measured by vaginal examination. A pessary of the diameter of about 1.5 cm less than this distance is usually selected. Two or three sizes near to that are kept ready.

Method of Introduction

Proper sized pessary is selected. The pessary is compressed between the thumb and index finger to introduce in the anteroposterior diameter of vagina. Then it is rotated in 90°. The upper circumference of the pessary fits into the posterior fornix while the lower circumference is pushed under the pubic symphysis.

After insertion, the patient is made to squat, walk around and cough. A correct sized pessary does not fall off nor does it produce any discomfort or pain due to overstretching of vagina.

Precautions for Pessary Users

- Daily vaginal douche by warm antiseptic is advisable to avoid infection.
- Pessary should be removed for cleaning and disinfecting before reintroduction every 2–3 months.
- Pessary should not be used for more than six months.

Disadvantages

- It does not cure prolapse. It only gives a temporary relief.
- Sloughing and ulceration of vagina due to pressure necrosis is known.
- Infection may result after prolonged use.
- Rarely a forgotten pessary may produce vesicovaginal fistula.
- It may get deeply embedded into the vagina.

RETROVERSION

Normally the uterus is anteverted and anteflexed. Sometimes it is in retroverted position.

Retrodisplacement is observed in almost 20% of the women but may not be pathological in all of them. Hence, mere finding of retroversion does not necessitate any surgical correction. Role of surgery for ventral suspension in cases of infertility and repeated early abortions is doubtful.

Nowadays, the indications for these procedures are limited. It is sometimes performed as a concurrent procedure at laparotomy done for any purpose in an infertile woman; e.g. tubal reconstructive surgery, myomectomy, ovariotomy, surgical excision of endometriotic patches, etc.

In such cases plication of round ligaments is performed. Both the round ligaments are shortened by plication by linen sutures taken from cornual ends to the lateral ends near internal inguinal ring.

8

Myomectomy

It is a surgical procedure in which uterine myomata are removed retaining the uterus for future child-bearing.

Indications

Presence of symptomatic uterine fibroids with:

a. Age less than 35 years
b. Patient anxious for conception
c. Infertility:
  • After exclusion of all other causes of infertility
  • Where there is potential relationship between size and location of tumour and infertility
d. Repeated spontaneous abortions or preterm deliveries in the absence of any other cause

An asymptomatic myoma less than 10–12 weeks size may be left alone under observation.

Contraindications

• Associated uterine or ovarian malignancies
• Associated blocked tubes and/or other causes of infertility.

Time of Surgery

Postmenstrual phase since:

a. Congestion is minimum
b. No risk of disturbing an early pregnancy

Myomectomy should never be performed during caesarean section for the risk of profuse haemorrhage.

Preoperative Considerations

a. Thorough evaluation of the couple for infertility
b. Preoperative USG, hysteroscopy and HSG to note the number, size and location of the tumours.
c. Preoperative medical therapy with Danazol or GnRH analogues reduces the size and vascularity significantly.
d. Prior consent for hysterectomy in case of uncontrollable haemorrhage.
e. Arrangements for blood transfusion.

Instruments

• Bonney's myomectomy clamp
• Instruments for laparotomy and hysterectomy.

Operative Principles

a. Evaluation of location and size of the tumours
b. Haemostasis
   • Bonney's clamp is used to occlude uterine arteries temporarily, which is released every 20 minutes. Alternatively, a rubber catheter can be used.
   • Infundibulopelvic ligaments are compressed by sponge holding forceps to occlude ovarian vessels.
   • Local infiltration of vasopressor agents
   • Swift surgical enucleation.
   • Obliteration of dead space in the residual cavity.
c. Incision
   • Number of incisions should be kept minimum for removal of all myomata.
   • Anterior midline incision on the uterus usually taken
   • Small myomata are removed through secondary tunneling incisions.
   • Bonny's hood for large posterior wall or fundal myoma
d. Cavity should be opened to remove submucous myomata.
e. Microsurgical principles should be followed.
f. Uterus should be maintained in anteverted position by some procedure for ventral suspension.

Small submucous myomata can be resected hysteroscopically; thus avoiding major surgery and scar on the uterus. The hospital stay is reduced.

Complications
Immediate
a. *Profuse primary haemorrhage:* A life saving hysterectomy may be required for uncontrolled haemorrhage.
b. *Injury to bladder or ureter:* Common with broad ligament and cervical myoma.
c. Infection

Delayed
a. *Recurrence of myoma:* To avoid this all the seedlings should be removed. Myomectomy undertaken after 30 years of age is less likely to be followed by recurrence.
b. Persistence of menorrhagia
   - Due to overlooked submucous myoma
   - Endometrial hyperplasia
c. Possibility of scar rupture in subsequent pregnancy if endometrial cavity was opened at the time of myomectomy.

Subsequent Pregnancy
Elective caesarean section if:
- Endometrial cavity was opened during myomectomy
- Infection had complicated the postoperative period
- Elderly primigravida
- Any other obstetric/medical complication.

Otherwise vaginal delivery can be allowed, as the myomectomy scar being on the non-pregnant uterus; usually heals well.

CERVICAL FIBROIDS
- Cervical fibroid is usually impacted in the pelvis with the uterine body sitting on the top.

- Myomectomy for cervical fibroid is rather difficult with increased risk of injury to bladder and ureter. Hence, preoperative IVP is necessary.
- Bonny's myomectomy clamp cannot be applied.

Anterior Cervical Myoma

Anterior cervical myoma displaces the urinary bladder in the abdomen necessitating extra care to avoid bladder injury while opening the abdomen. For removal of such myoma a transverse incision is taken between the two round ligaments deviding the peritoneum. Bladder is pushed down. Capsule is incised vertically or transversely and the tumour is enucleated.

Posterior Cervical Myoma

Vertical incision is taken through the loose peritoneum covering the tumour.

Central Cervical Myoma

Uterus is bisected before enucleation of the tumour. It is necessary to define the cervical canal before suturing the uterus.

Lateral Cervical Myoma

It displaces the ureter. Operative technique is difficult.

BROAD LIGAMENT MYOMA

a. *True broad ligament myoma:* Arises from the broad ligament itself. Ureter runs on the inner side and below it.
b. *False broad ligament myoma:* It is a uterine myoma growing from the lateral wall of the uterus. It displaces the uterine vessels and ureter laterally.
   - Risk of injury to ureter high, preoperative IVP to reduce the risk
   - Enucleation of the tumour by incising the overlying peritoneum.

9   Ovarian Surgery

OVARIAN CYSTECTOMY

It is a procedure for enucleation of a cyst in the ovary.

The capsule of the cyst is incised and the cyst is enucleated by its gentle dissection from the capsule. The redundant capsule is excised and the raw area is closed with fine catgut after achieving haemostasis.

Simple serous cyst, dermoid cyst, etc. can be removed in this manner.

Advantage
The normal ovarian tissue left behind continues its function of ovulation and hormone production.

OVARIOTOMY

Removal of the entire ovary along with cyst or tumour in it.

Indications

- Benign ovarian neoplasms where normal ovarian tissue can not be identified.
- Twisted ovarian cyst.

Advantage
Easy and quick surgical procedure.

Disadvantage
If in future the other ovary becomes pathological needing its removal, the patient looses both ovaries and reaches her menopause at a premature age.

OOPHORECTOMY

Surgical removal of apparently normal ovary.

Indications

i. When an ovary is severely involved in extraovarian tumour, cyst, adhesions or endometriosis and cannot be retained easily.
ii. *Along with hysterectomy:*
   • All postmenopausal patients
   • Premenopausal patients with genital tract malignancies
   • When ovarian blood supply is severely compromised
iii. *Carcinoma breast:* When the tumour is oestrogen dependent. However, currently antioestrogens are used in such cases.

Procedure

Surgical removal of the ovary is achieved by clamping, dividing and transfixing the infundibulopelvic ligament along with ovarian vessels laterally and ovariouterine ligament medially.

PROPHYLACTIC PREMENOPAUSAL OOPHORECTOMY AT HYSTERECTOMY

Eliminates the possibility of future risk of ovarian malignancy; which is not more than 0.1% to 0.2%.

Disadvantages
• Sudden menopausal syndrome
• Increased risk of subsequent development of osteoporosis, hypertension and ischaemic heart disease.

LAPAROSCOPIC MULTIPLE PUNCTURES OF THE CYSTS WITH ELECTROCAUTERY OR LASER

Laparoscopic ovarian drilling is performed in cases of anovulatory infertility due to polycystic ovarian disease where medical management has failed. Electrocautery or laser is used. Up to 15 punctures are made on each side. Ovaries are lavaged with normal saline which reduces the risk of adhesion formation.

Surgery restores the endocrine milieu (decrease in serum levels of LH, androgenic steroids and LH/FSH ratio) and improves fertility over a year.

Advantages
- One time treatment.
- Monitoring not required
- Ovulation occurs in 80% and pregnancy in 60–70%

Disadvantages
- Risk of pelvic adhesions which can reduce the fertility.
- Rarely premature ovarian failure
- Risk of laparoscopy and anesthesia

Comment
In past, a wedge of ovarian tissue was removed at laparotomy to reduce the volume of androgen producing tissue. Post-operative intrapelvic adhesions were common. Laparoscopic ovarian drilling has replaced this procedure as it has less adhesion formation and similar results in correction of endocrine abnormalities.

10 | Urinary Incontinence

Urinary incontinence is involuntary leakage of urine.

Varieties

1. *Stress incontinence:* This is urinary incontinence on straining; which may be due to:
   - Genuine stress incontinence
   - Detrusor instability
2. *Overflow incontinence:* Mostly due to neurological causes
3. *True incontinence:* This is continuous leakage of urine; which may be due to:
   - Fistulae
   - Congenital abnormalities–ectopic ureter
4. *Functional incontinence*

   In true incontinence bladder is empty while in overflow incontinence the bladder is overdistended.

GENUINE STRESS INCONTINENCE

In this condition, there is involuntary loss of urine when the intra-abdominal pressure exceeds the maximal urethral pressure without detrusor activity.

Multiparity, genital prolapse, menopausal atrophy and previous bladder neck surgery can predispose to this condition which is due to weakness of urethral sphincter mechanism and descent of bladder neck; and not due to bladder abnormality.

Surgical Treatment

When the patient has cystourethrocoele, this condition can be cured surgically by plication of the paraurethral and paravesical fascia to elevate the posterior urethra and urethrovesical junction to a high retropubic (intra-abdominal) position. This can be achieved by:

- Anterior colporrhaphy
- Kelley's stitch

When the condition exists without cystourethrocoele, or previous repair of cystourethrocoele has failed to give relief; retropubic suspension procedures are carried out.

In nulliparous postmenopausal woman having loss of urogenital diaphragm, mild incontinence may be relieved by vaginal procedures; while in severe cases retropubic suspension may be required.

Preoperative Evaluation

1. *Physical Examination*

- Condition of bladder–distended or empty
- Cystourethrocoele
- Vaginal length and mobility
- *Bonney's test:* After testing for the incontinence, right index and middle fingers are pressed firmly upwards in the lateral urethral recesses to elevate and support the region of the bladder neck. The patient is asked to cough. If incontinence is controlled with this maneuver, it indicates that the surgical repair will relieve the incontinence.
- Complete neurological examination

2. *Urine Examination*

To exclude infection
- Urine analysis
- Culture and sensitivity

3. *Cystoscopy*

To exclude local organic lesions

4. *Urodynamic Evaluation* (Table 10.1)

To exclude detrusor overactivity. Helps to detect the intrinsic sphincter deficiency and helps to choose the correct surgery.

The Aims of Surgery

1. Elevate the bladder neck; i.e. urethrovesical junction into the abdominal zone of pressure so that there is always a positive pressure gradient between the higher closure pressure of the urethra and the bladder (positive closure pressure).
2. Support the bladder neck to prevent its funneling or opening in response to a rise in intravesical pressure.
3. Increase urethral or outlet resistance without producing obstruction.

Anterior Colporrhaphy

- Traditionally used vaginal operation for women having cystocele and stress urinary incontinence (SUI).
- Kelley's bladder neck suture is put.
- Buttressing of the bladder neck and bladder is done by approximating pubocervical fascia across them.

Advantages
- Quicker method
- Can correct genital prolapse simultaneousely
- Cure rate around 60%
- Postoperative period smooth

Effective elevation of bladder neck is not possible with this operation. In view of the poor long-term success rates it is not recommended for treatment of SUI.

Modified Burch Colposuspension

- Entry into retropubic space abdominally through extraperi-toneal approach
- Supravaginal fascia of the lateral vaginal fornices is sutured by three pairs of sutures to the ipsilateral iliopectineal ligaments as follows: First: below the bladder neck, second: at the bladder neck and third at higher level.

Advantages
- Correction of cystourethrocoele possible
- *High cure rate:* Primary procedure 96%; secondary procedure 76%

Disadvantage

Adequate elevation is not possible when vaginal capacity and mobility is decreased due to previous surgery, scarring or menopausal atrophy.

Complications
- *Early:* Bleeding

  Damage to bladder, urethra, bowel, vessels
- *Delayed:* Voiding dysfunction and detrusor overactivity, enterocele may occur.

Laparoscopic colposuspension
- Less invasive, less hospital stay
- Higher complication rates
- Lesser long term cure rates

  With availability of minimally invasive midurethral slings this approach is not being used.

Suprapubic Sling Operations

Conventional sling procedures are complicated procedures in which the sling is placed under the urethrovesical junction.
- Vaginal and abdominal incisions are required to insert the sling
- Two varieties of slings can be used:
  - *Autogenous tissue:* Fascia lata, rectus sheath fascia

    Disadvantage: Variation in tensile strength
  - *Inorganic substances:* Mersilene, nylon, marlex

    Disadvantages: Foreign body reaction, infection and sinus formation
- Experience is necessary for adjusting correct tension on the sling.
  - Too much tension can lead to retention of urine, ulceration of urethra
  - Too less tension is associated with recurrence of incontinence.
- These procedures are usually reserved for recurrent stress incontinence.

Midurethral Slings: *Tension Free Vaginal Tape (TVT)*

Polypropylene mesh is placed tension free under the mid-urethra via vaginal approach exiting abdominally through the retropubic space. Cure rates up to 84 to 100% reported. Effectiveness is similar to colposuspension.

Several modifications of the procedure have been suggested to minimize the injuries to vessels, bowel, urinary tract. Trans opturator placement of sling from outside in or passing the sling from inside out has been shown to have similar cure rates with less injuries to urinary tract.

Needle Suspension Procedures: (Pareyra, Stamey)

The operations involved suspending sutures from vaginal, paravaginal or paraurethral tissues to the anterior abdominal wall with an objective of elevating the bladder neck.

These procedures were simple, requiring less operating time, and less hospital stay. However, they had more complications (infection, rejection of sutures, vesical stone formation, etc.) and very high failure rates. Hence, these are not recommended.

DETRUSOR OVERACTIVITY

In this, the urethral function is unaffected, but the bladder contracts in an uninhibited fashion. Intravesical pressure exceeds the urethral pressure leading to incontinence.

Etiology

- Secondary to upper motor neurone lesions; e.g. multiple sclerosis
- Idiopathic

Symptoms

- Urge incontinence
- Nocturia
- Enuresis
- Stress urinary incontinence

The diagnosis is confirmed by cystometry. Medications used for treatment include anticholinergic drugs (Oxybutynin).

OVERFLOW INCONTINENCE

Any condition of chronic retention of urine leads to overflow incontinence. Intravesical pressure exceeds maximum urethral pressure due to bladder distension; but often in absence of detrusor activity.

Etiology

- Urethral obstruction
- Detrusor inactivity
- Upper or lower motor neurone lesions
- Drugs-ganglion blockers, anticholinergic drugs, β-adrenergic stimulants, tricyclic antidepressants
- Epidural anaesthesia
- Surgery
- Pelvic mass
- Inflammation of urethra, vulva or vagina
- Prolonged catheterization

Diagnosis

Symptoms

- Constant dribbling incontinence
- Stress incontinence

On Examination

Distended bladder noted

Cystometry

- Delayed first sensation to void
- Large bladder capacity
- Unusually *flat* detrusor muscle trace

URINARY FISTULAE
Common Types and Etiology

1. Vesicovaginal (VVF)
   - Obstetric injury → Pressure necrosis following obstructed labour due to the impacted head in

Table 10.1: Urodynamic indicators

Urodynamic indications	Normal	Stress incontinence	Detrusor overactivity	Overflow
Maximum urethral pressure	> Intravesical	< Intravesical	Intravesical++	Intravesical++
Residual urine volume	<100	Normal	Normal	Large
First voiding sensation at (ml)	120–200	Normal	Early	Absent
Strong desire to voide (5 ml)	450–600	Normal	250	Absent
Intravesical pressure rise on bladder filling (cm of water)	15	15	>20 up to 60	Higher
Contraction trace	Normal	Normal	Overactivity	Flat

midpelvis. Manifests 5–7 days after injury.

→ Direct injury during obstetrical operations, manifests immediately.

- Surgical trauma → Hysterectomy, caesarean section, colporrhaphy, etc.
- Malignancy → Carcinoma cervix
- Radiation → Radiation necrosis
- Infection → Tuberculosis
- Traumatic → Foreign body
  → Accidental

2. Ureterovaginal: Surgical injuries
3. Urethrovaginal
4. Vesicocervical

Diagnostic Tests and Preoperative Evaluation

Three Swabs Test

- Three tampoons are placed in the vagina.
- Dilute solution of methylene blue is instilled into the bladder through a catheter.
- Patient is made to walk around for 10–15 minutes.
- Tampoons are removed and examined.

Findings	Interpretation
– Lowest tampoon soaked and blue	Urethral leakage
– Middle or upper tampoon soaked and blue	VVF
– Upper tampoon soaked but not blue	Ureteral fistula

Cystoscopy

To confirm:

- Size and position of fistula
- Relation of fistula to ureteral orifices and vesical sphincter
- Possibility of more than one fistula
- Urinary spurt from ureteric orifice. If there is no spurt due to obstruction, then ureteric catheterisation helps to locate the level of obstruction.

Intravenous Pyelography

- To exclude hydroureter, hydronephrosis.
- **Biopsy** from edge of the fistula if malignancy is suspected.

Preoperative

Excoriation of skin, if present, is to be treated preoperatively by application of topical soothening agent like vaseline.

Prevention

- Avoiding difficult forceps
- Timely caesarean section
- Prolonged catheterisation following obstructed labour with haematuria
- Avoiding bladder injury during surgery
- Immediate recognition and proper repair of bladder injury during surgery.

Initial Treatment

Continuous catheterisation for:
- Spontaneous healing of small fistulae
- Minimising the size of fistula
- Preventing the tissue excoriation due to leakage of urine.

Surgical Closure

Time of Surgery

Six months after the causative event, but not earlier than 2–3 months.

Three Approaches

Vaginal, transperitoneal extravesical, transvesical

Vaginal Repair

Vaginal approach is always preferred. Usually, flap splitting technique with repair in layers is performed.

Principles

- Adequate exposure of fistula. Incision is taken 1 cm above and below the fistula, and encircling it.
- Excision of the fistula tract
- Excision of all scar tissue
- Wide mobilisation of the vaginal mucosa
- Use of 3/0 delayed absorbable suture material, i.e. vicryl on fine atraumatic needle for bladder mucosa
- Covering layers through bladder muscularis–3/0 interrupted sutures are taken. The sutures should be without tension.
- Vagina is closed in a vertical manner by interrupted sutures without tension on them.
- *Bladder drainage:* Urethral or suprapubic catheter for 2 weeks. During postoperative period, catheter patency must be checked. Suction drainage may be employed to keep the bladder completely empty.

Transperitoneal Extravesical Repair

This approach is selected in cases of:
a. High fistula
b. Fistula closer to ureter
c. Previous failed attempts of repair.

Principles

- Abdominal total hysterectomy is performed.
- Bladder and vagina are separated from each other by delicate dissection.
- Vaginal opening is closed separately.
- Bladder is closed in two layers.
- Suprapubic drainage is maintained.

Transvesical Repair

This approach is preferred in cases of:
  i. High fistula inaccessible vaginally
 ii. Failed previous attempts leading to scarring.

Principles
- Bladder is opened in the midline.
- Posteriorly incision is extended up to the fistula.
- Fistula is excised.
- Vagina is sutured.
- Bladder is closed.

Success of Fistula Repair
- Proper technique of repair
- Use of correct suture material
- Amount of scarring present due to number of previous repairs
- Infection
- Amount of tissue loss
- *Etiological factor:* Fistulae due to malignancy and radiation heal poorly.

Complications of Fistula Repair
- Ureteric obstruction
- Haemorrhage
- Urinary infection
- Failed repair

URINARY TRACT INJURIES (DURING GYNAECOLOGICAL SURGERY)

Bladder and ureter are likely to sustain injury in almost every Gynaecological surgical procedure. The factors predisposing to such injuries are:
- Repeat caesarean section or previous laparotomy scar
- Tumours destroying the anatomical relationship, e.g. cervical or broad ligament fibroids
- Radical surgery involving extensive dissection of ureter and separation of bladder
- Obesity
- Malignant infiltration
- Cases of prolonged obstructed labour with oedematous bladder

- Dense adhesions due to extensive endometriosis or pelvic inflammatory disease
- Poor technical skill

The injury can result due to
- Cutting the bladder or ureter by sharp instrument during dissection
- Clamping and suturing them inadvertantly in ligature
- Striping the ureter extensively of its sheath affecting its blood supply leading to avascular necrosis of ureter.

BLADDER INJURY
Risk of Bladder Injury

i. While opening the peritoneal cavity

   Prevention
   - Empty the bladder before surgery
   - Catheter retained in bladder during surgery
   - Careful opening of peritoneum under vision at higher level of incision

ii. While separating the bladder away from the cervix by vigorous blunt dissection.

iii. While closing the vaginal opening during hysterectomy, bladder may be included in the suture line.

iv. While suturing the caesarean incision or closing visceral peritoneum on the uterus, vesical angle may be included.

v. During vaginal surgery, while dissecting the bladder and opening the vesicouterine pouch of the peritoneum.

Treatment

- Suturing the rent in bladder by 3/0 vicryl or catgut in two layers
- Postoperative continuous drainage of bladder by self-retaining catheter for 7–10 days
- Use of antibiotics

INJURIES TO URETER
Risks and Sites

- While clamping infundibulopelvic ligament during hysterectomy
- While ligating and dividing the uterine arteries
- While clamping the cardinal ligaments
- While closing the pelvic peritoneum
- During internal iliac ligation
- During surgery for cervical or broad ligament tumours.

Nature of Injury

Division, crushing, inclusion in the ligature, avascular necrosis.

Prevention

In difficult cases, where ureteric injury is anticipated
- Preoperative intravenous pyelography
- Ureteric catheterisation before surgery
- Preoperative intravenous indigo carmine or methylene blue
- Intrafascial technique of hysterectomy.

Treatment

The treatment depends upon:
- Time lost between the injury and its recognition
- Site of injury

Injury Recognized during Surgery

1. *Injury within 4–5 cm from ureterovesical junction:* Implantation of the ureter into the bladder
2. *Injury in the region of pelvic brim:* The site being too high for implantation, uretero-ureteral anastomosis is performed.
3. *Ureteric damage within the lower half of broad ligament:* Psoas muscle hitch procedure–bladder is well mobilised widely and the dome is anchored to the psoas muscle near the pelvic brim. Then ureterovesical anastomosis is performed.
4. *Boari flap procedure:* Ureteric anastomosis to the bladder dome by rolling up a flap from bladder.

5. Large segment of the pelvic ureter is injured and only the upper half of the ureter is intact–transperitoneal anastomosis to the ureter on the opposite side.
6. Simple ligation of the ureter is done only in cases of advanced pelvic cancer where life expectancy is low. This leads to asymptomatic death of kidney in absence of infection. The other kidney must be functioning.
7. Skin ureterostomy can be tried as a last resort.

Injury Recognized Late

1. It leads to pyelitis, which is evident by loin pain and unexplained fever. Tender mass is ballotable in the loin due to hydronephrosis.
2. May lead to ureterovaginal fistula.
3. Postoperative IVP is useful for diagnosis.
4. If unilateral hydronephrosis or unilateral impairment of kidney function is noted then cystoscopy and ureteric catheterisation is performed.
   a. *Catheter can bypass the obstruction:* It should be left in place for 14 days.
   b. *Catheter cannot bypass the obstruction:* Immediate ureteral repair or percutaneous nephrostomy followed by surgical repair after 6–8 weeks.

Delayed surgical repair is performed when
- Patient has undergone extensive dissection in a surgical procedure.
- In presence of infection
- In debilitated patient with poor healing capacity
- Where the injury has taken place near the pelvic brim.

11

Congenital Malformations

CREATION OF ARTIFICIAL VAGINA
Indication
Congenital absence of vagina

Timing
Prior to marriage

Methods
Nonsurgical
Intermittent pressure

Surgical
- McIndoe operation
- William's vulvovaginoplasty

1. McINDOE OPERATION
- Dissection of adequate space between bladder and rectum
- Split-thickness skin grafting over a mould

Human amnion can be used instead of skin graft
Continuous and prolonged dilatation of artificially created vagina by using a mould.

Mould
Wooden mould having anterior groove for urethra is commonly used. Alternatively plastic or sialastic mould can be used.

Complications

- Injury to bladder, urethra or rectum
- Haemorrhage
- Failure to take up the graft
- Stricture

2. WILLIAM'S VULVOVAGINOPLASTY

- Horseshoe shaped incision is taken in the vulva, which extends across the perineum and along the medial side of labia to the level of external urethral meatus.
- Edges of skin are mobilised.
- Inner skin margins are sutured together.
- Second layer of suture is taken to approximate subcutaneous fat and perineal muscles for support.
- Outer skin margins are approximated.

By this method, a pouch accommodating two fingers up to the depth of 3 cm is possible.

Follow-up

Three weeks later vagina is dilated by vaginal dilators.

Advantage

Simple and safe method without any postoperative pain and with speedy recovery.

Disadvantage

Vagina is constructed with unusual angle.

METROPLASTY

Surgical procedures for unification of congenital uterine malformations like septate or bicornuate uterus.

Indications

- Habitual abortions or repeated preterm deliveries due to uterine anomaly.
- Primary infertility, after all other factors have been excluded.

Preoperative Evaluation

- *Hysterography:* Cannot differentiate between septate and bicornuate uterus.
- *Hysteroscopy:* Can visualize the septum.
- *Ultrasonography:* Can help in noting the external contour. However, by itself, it may not be diagnostic.
- *Laparoscopy:* Can visualize the external contour of the uterus and diagnose bicornuate uterus, but not septate uterus. Can diagnose arcuate uterus, unicornuate uterus and rudimentary horn of a bicornuate uterus which is not communicating with the cervix.

Thus, all the diagnostic aids are complimentary to each other in confirming the nature of the anomaly.

Surgical Techniques

1. Strassman Operation

This procedure is used for unification of bicornuate uterus.

- Uterine cornue are incised on their medial sides longitudinally to open the endometrial cavities.
- The myometrium is approximated in two layers. The anterior edges and the posterior edges sutured with interrupted figure of eight sutures with 3/0 vicryl.

2. Jone's Operation

This is performed for septate uterus.

- Anteroposterior incision is taken on either side of the midline until the uterine cavity is reached.
- Wedge of septum is excised carefully avoiding damage to fallopian tubes.
- Endocervical canal is checked for patency.
- Myometrium is sutured with interrupted 3/0 vicryl sutures. Both anterior and posterior edges are approximated respectively starting from below upwards.
- Serosal layer is sutured separately.

3. Tompkin's Operation

This is an alternative method suggested for cases with septate uterus.

- Single median incision is taken to divide the uterine corpus and septum.
- The incision is deepened to open the uterine cavity.
- Each half is then incised. No septal tissue is removed.
- The myometrium is reapproximated in two layers.

4. Hysteroscopic Resection of Septum

A thin septum can be resected hysteroscopically; under laparoscopic control. This avoids major abdominal surgery.

Complications

- *Haemorrhage:* This can be minimized by using tourniquet around the cervix to compress the uterine vessels.
- Fallopian tubes may be damaged if extensive wedge is excised.
- Cervix may get damaged or endocervical canal may get blocked.
- Infection
- *Intrauterine adhesions:* IUCD may be inserted to prevent this.

Obstetrics

12. Surgical Evacuation
13. Cervical Encerclage
14. Prenatal Diagnosis
15. Version
16. Episiotomy
17. Instrumental Vaginal Delivery
18. Caesarean Section
19. Obstetric Haemorrhage
20. Destructive Operations
21. Manual Removal of Placenta

Surgical Evacuation

This is a commonly performed operation in obstetrics for emptying the uterus of the products of conception.

Indications

a. Inevitable abortion
b. Incomplete abortion
c. Missed abortion
d. Vesicular mole
e. First trimester MTP

The evacuation is safely carried out for abortion cases when the uterine size is smaller than 12 weeks size. However, for vesicular mole even larger uterus can be evacuated surgically with suction.

Instruments

- Complete set of D and C instruments, ovum forceps
- Suction cannulae with suction machine or MVA syringe and cannulae.

Methods

1. Instrumental evacuation
2. *Vacuum aspiration:* Electrical or manual (vide MTP)

A. INEVITABLE AND INCOMPLETE ABORTIONS

In these cases, internal os of the cervix is already dilated; hence procedure can be performed without anaesthesia. Only parenteral premedication is administered.

Procedure

1. Cervix is visualized and its anterior lip is grasped by sponge holding forceps. Since pregnant cervix is very soft, traumatic instrument like volsellum is not to be used.
2. Ovum forceps is introduced into the uterine cavity in closed fashion, opened inside to grasp the products of conception and then it is turned through 90° to ensure that the uterine wall is not caught in it. Then it is withdrawn out. This procedure is repeated till all the bits of conceptus are removed.
3. Finally, the cavity is curetted by blunt curette. The evacuated products should be sent for histopathological study to rule out vesicular mole.
   Antibiotics are administered.

Complications

1. Uterine perforation
2. Incomplete evacuation with persistent vaginal bleeding
3. Infection

B. MISSED ABORTION

It is a condition with prolonged retention of dead foetus. Cervical dilatation and vacuum aspiration is done under LA/GA if uterine size is less than 12 weeks. The pregnancy can be terminated by medical methods also.

Special Preoperative Preparations

1. *Study of coagulation profile of the patient:* Bleeding time, clotting time, platelet count, clot retraction time, prothrombin time, serum fibrinogen degradation products.
2. Fresh blood should be cross-matched and kept ready as there is risk of disseminated intravascular coagulopathy leading to profuse bleeding due to retained dead conceptus.
   Antibiotics are administered.

C. VESICULAR MOLE

Vacuum aspiration under general anaesthesia is the method of choice irrespective of the size of uterus. Gentle curettage is done in the end and the sample is sent for histopathological examination. Intraoperative sonography may be useful for avoiding perforation and confirming that the uterus is empty. Medical methods of pregnancy termination are avoided for fear of trophoblastic embolization.

Preoperative Preparation
Blood should be cross-matched and kept ready.

Complications
Immediate
- Profuse bleeding
- Perforation
- Infection
- Retained molar tissue

Delayed
- Persistent trophoblastic disease
- Choriocarcinoma

Postoperative Care
- Adequate blood replacement
- Antibiotics
- There is no need for routine second curettage
- Baseline investigations like X-ray chest and serum β-HCG levels at discharge
- Reliable contraception

Follow-up
- Prevent pregnancy for a period of 6 months by using reliable method of contraception. Conception may be allowed after serum β-HCG levels remain normal for 6 months.
- Combined oral contraceptive pills may be used for effective contraception. Barrier methods of contraception may be preferred until β-HCG levels revert to normal.

- IUD is not advised on account of irregular vaginal bleeding often experienced with.
- Periodic systematic follow-up for early detection of gestational trophoblastic neoplasia is very important. During this follow-up careful clinical examination and serum β-HCG estimation is done. The clinical examination should include looking for:
  - i. Abnormal vaginal bleeding
  - ii. Enlarged soft uterus
  - iii. Evidence of metastasis in lungs (cough, haemoptysis), brain and anterior vaginal wall

  β-HCG levels are done every 2 weeks till it falls to normal level, monthly for 6 months thereafter. If it remains normal for 6 months then follow-up is discontinued and pregnancy is allowed.

Chemotherapy is indicated if

- The serum β-HCG remain static (platwau) or shows a rise after a fall
- Serum β-HCG remains detectable for 6 months or more
- Histological diagnosis of choriocarcinoma

Prophylactic methotrexate therapy is not recommended routinely and may be considered in high-risk complete moles if follow-up with HCG estimation is not possible.

13 | Cervical Encerclage

This is surgical reinforcement of the incompetent cervix.

Indication
Incompetent internal os of the cervix.

Diagnosis during Pregnancy
- H/o repeated midtrimester spontaneous abortions, which are rapid, relatively painless, usually preceeded by leaking and expulsion of live foetus.
- *Serial USG:* Progressively dilating internal os, decreasing cervical length, and membranes dipping into the cervical canal
- Serial vaginal examinations carried out fortnightly during pregnancy reveal progressive dilatation and effacement of the cervix.

Time of Operation
- At the diagnosis of the condition in second trimester.
- Prophylactically around 14th to 16th week of gestation.

Why not to be Performed in First Trimester?
- The first trimester abortions are usually due to germplasm defect and cervical encerclage cannot prevent them. Therefore, the procedure is carried out only when viable pregnancy is established.
- Cervical incompetence generally does not cause first trimester abortions.

Contraindications

- Rupture of membranes
- Uterine contractions
- Uterine bleeding
- Chorioamnionitis
- Cervix dilated >4 cm
- Polyhydramnios
- Dead foetus
- Abnormal foetus
- Lower genital tract infection

Anaesthesia

General anaesthesia

Preoperative

i. Ultrasonography to ensure live and normal foetus
ii. VDRL to exclude syphilis

McDONALD'S OPERATION

This is the simplified modification of Shirodkar's encerclage operation. Here, the reinforcement stitch is taken below the level of the internal os at cervicovaginal junction without any dissection of the urinary bladder.

Instruments

Right-angled retractor, half circle nontraumatic suturing needle, suture material–braided black silk no. 1 or 2 or thick monofilament nylon.

Steps of Operation

1. Cervix is exposed and the anterior lip of the cervix is held by sponge holding forceps.
2. A purse string suture is taken starting anteriorly and taking four bites through the substance of the cervical tissue.
3. Knots of the two ends of the suture material are tied anterior to the cervix taking care not to tie them too tightly.

Removal of the Stitch

At 38 weeks of gestation or at the onset of labour–whichever is earlier.

Postoperative Care

- Rest in head low position to avoid pressure of foetal head on internal os
- Prophylactic tocolytic drugs like Isoxuprine, Salbutamol
- Sedation
  Patient can be discharged after the uterus has relaxed completely.

Instructions

- Extra rest, preferably in head low position
- Avoid lifting heavy weights
- No travelling
- Fortnightly antenatal check up
- Continuation of tocolytic agents orally if indicated, particularly if the uterus shows signs of irritability.

Complications

1. Accidental Rupture of Membranes

In such case, the abortion becomes inevitable. This can be prevented by taking care not to encroach into cervical canal during the procedure.

2. Uterine Contractions

Which can be prevented by:

- Avoiding the operative procedure till uterus is completely relaxed.
- Avoiding too much of manipulation.
- Strict bedrest in head low position postoperatively.
- Timely use of tocolytic agents, if the uterus becomes irritable.

3. Failure to Prevent Obstetric Mishaps

- If diagnosis is incorrect

- If done too late when membranes are bulging. In such cases, the membranes can be pushed up giving head low position overnight and by pushing them gently with either a gauze piece soaked in normal saline or by Foley's catheter balloon
- If performed when the uterus is contracting.

4. Infection

This can be prevented by proper case selection and following disinfection procedures.

SHIRODKAR'S OPERATION

This is the original operation devised by late Dr. VN Shirodkar from Mumbai. It comprises strengthening the internal os of the cervix with the help of mersilene tape.

Instruments

- Sim's/Auvard's speculum, anterior vaginal wall rectractor, sponge holding forceps, right-angled retractors, B.P. Handle no. 4 with blade no. 22
- Special aneurism needles–right-sided and left-sided (they are mirror images of each other)
- Mersilene tape, needle holder, scissors, catgut no. 1/0 on needle.

Steps of Operation

1. Patient's legs are tied in lithotomy position.
2. The cervix is exposed with the help of Sim's/Auvard's speculum.
3. Anterior lip of the cervix is held with sponge holding forceps.
4. Transverse incision of about 2 cm length is taken at cervico-vaginal junction in the anterior vaginal wall.
5. The bladder is pushed up with finger and gauze dissection.
6. The internal os is identified by the attachments of the bladder pillars.

7. Shirodkar's special aneurism needle is passed submucosally on one side through the incision and brought out posteriorly to the cervix at 6 O'clock position by taking a vertical nick. Mersilene tape is threaded in the tip and the needle is brought back along with the tape.

8. The needle is introduced similarly submucosally on the other side and the tape is threaded in its tip. The needle is brought out posteriorly through the same posterior incision to bring the tape posteriorly and the needle is removed.

9. The two ends of the tape are tied posteriorly.

10. Both incisions are closed by few interrupted catgut sutures.

At term mersilene tape can be divided and the patient can be delivered vaginally.

Dr. VN Shirodkar, in his original operation used a strip of fascia lata when it was obligatory to leave it permanently and effect the delivery by caesarean section. For comparison of two cerclage procedures *see* Table 13.1.

Table 13.1: Comparison of Shirodkar's and McDonald's cervical encerclage

Shirodkar's	*McDonald's*
• Original surgery	• Modification of Shirodkar's operation
• Technically skillful	• Technically easy
• Requires more time	• Requires less time
• More operative bleeding	• No operative bleeding
• Suture material–Mersilene tape–costly	• Suture material–Breaded black silk or monofilament nylon–much lower cost
• Special Shirodkar's encerclage needle required	• Oridnary nontraumatic curved suturing needle to be used
• Knot posteriorly	• Knot anteriorly
• Length of cervix does not put limitations on procedure. Indicated when cervix is short, amputated or torn	• Cannot be performed in too short cervix (congenital or amputated), and extensive cervical tears where reaching above the apex of the tear is not possible

WURM PROCEDURE

This is a procedure of cervical reinforcement suggested for the treatment of cervical incompetence with effaced cervix. The suture material used is braided silk no. 3. A stitch is inserted through cervical os from positions 12 O'clock to 6 O'clock and back to 12 O'clock position. Another stitch is taken at right angles to this at positions starting from 3 O'clock to 9 O'clock and back to 3 O'clock position. The entry and exit points are approximately separated from each other by 1 cm distance; thus cervical tissue of 1 cm each is incorporated at 12, 3, 6 and 9 O'clock positions respectively.

TRANSABDOMINAL ENCERCLAGE

This is abdominal approach for encerclage of the incompetent os of the cervix where vaginal encerclage is not possible due to too short cervix.

Indications

- Congenitally short cervix
- Amputated cervix
- Marked scarring of the cervix.

Procedure

Mersilene strand stitch is taken to encircle the isthmial region around 14 weeks of gestation. Elective caesarean section is done at term and the stitch is left in situ for the future pregnancies.

Advantage
Since the stitch is left in situ, no need to undergo encerclage operation during every pregnancy.

Disadvantage
Since vaginal delivery is not possible in these cases, it involves two major surgical procedures–the abdominal encirclage and the caesarean section.

NONSURGICAL MANAGEMENT
Use of Pessary

Vitsky had suggested use of Hodge Smith pessary, which would change the inclination of the cervical canal and redistribute the weight of the growing conceptus. Advanced cases, where encirclage is not possible, may be treated by this management.

PRECONCEPTIONAL MANAGEMENT
Diagnosis

- Typical obstetric history of repeated midtrimester abortions.
- *Dilator test (Snap test):* Hegar's dilator no. 8 can be introduced easily without any resistance. Also while withdrawing it, no characteristic snapping closure is felt.
- *Hysterography:* Funneling seen at the isthmus with the width of more than 8 mm at the internal os. Hysterography may be performed in midluteal phase for this purpose.

Place of the Preconceptional Encerclage

Not performed as:
- Cannot judge the extent of tightness required, hence may become very tight or may remain loose.
- Unexplained infertility is known after cervical encerclage done in a nonpregnant state.

14

Prenatal Diagnosis

Prenatal diagnosis of foetal diseases is now possible with modern techniques. Decisions about therapeutic termination of pregnancy or foetal therapy can be based on findings of such study.

Diagnosis of foetal maturity, chromosomal and other foetal abnormalities and foetal anaemia in Rh incompatibility are some of the areas of prenatal diagnosis.

The procedures for prenatal diagnosis are:
1. Ultrasonography
2. Amniocentesis
3. Chorion villus sampling
4. Cordocentesis–foetal blood sampling
5. Foetoscopy
6. Foetal tissue biopsy

ULTRASONOGRAPHY

Indications

First Trimester

- Early diagnosis of pregnancy
  - At 5 weeks, the identification of intrauterine gestational sac as anechoic structure having highly echogenic border
  - At 7th or 8th week, foetal pole can be visualized and the cardiac pulsations can be seen.
- Impending abortion
  - Poorly formed or sagging gestational sac
  - Decrease in decidual reaction around the sac
  - Subchorionic bleed
  - Sac low in the uterus

- Incomplete abortion: Retained products of conception
- Nonviable pregnancy
  - Before 8 weeks:
    - ♦ Irregular crenate sac
  - After 8 weeks
    - ♦ Blighted ovum–large empty gestational sac
    - ♦ Small for dates gestational sac
    - ♦ Absence of foetal heart activity
- Ectopic pregnancy
  - Empty uterus in spite of positive β-HCG test
  - Normal to slightly enlarged uterus
  - Well-developed adnexal gestational sac
  - Diffusely echogenic adnexal mass representing haemato-salpinx or blood in the adnexa or pouch of Douglas
- Molar pregnancy shows multiple small echogenic areas giving a 'snow storm' appearance
- Uterine abnormalities

Second Trimester

- Cervical incompetence
- Foetal malformations can be detected by 18th week
- Cardiac anomalies are seen about 20–22 weeks
- Foetal biometry
- Placental localization
- Multiple pregnancy
  - Detection of
    - ♦ Abnormal growth of foeti
    - ♦ Congenital malformations
    - ♦ Conjoint twins
    - ♦ Discordant twins
  - Monochorionic and dichorionic twins by the thickness of dividing membrane and appearance at the membrane–placenta interface.

Third Trimester
- Foetal growth monitoring and detection of IUGR
- Assessment of foetal well-being in complicated pregnancies helps in deciding timing of delivery, significant alerts being
  - Manning's score <= 6, amniotic fluid index <5
- Foetal death
  - Absence of foetal heart activity and foetal movement
  - Foetal oedema
- *Foetal presentation:* When clinically uncertain
- Polyhydramnios
- Estimation of foetal weight

AMNIOCENTESIS

It is a procedure in which amniotic sac is punctured to aspirate amniotic fluid.

Indications

Diagnostic aspiration

1. *Maturity of Foetal Lungs*
- Lecithin–sphingomyelin ratio >2
- Bubble stability test (shake test) positive
- Presence of phosphatidylglycerol.

2. *Amniotic Fluid Bilirubin Concentration*
- *Rh negative sensitized mother in third trimester:* To know the severity of foetal haemolytic disease and also for planning intrauterine transfusion or the delivery.
- It also indicates foetal maturity although it is a less sensitive test.

3. *Genetic Disorders*

α-Fetoproteins concentration in amniotic fluid is measured in second trimester (16 to 20 weeks) in cases showing raised maternal serum AFP. It is considerably elevated in:
- Open neural tube defects, e.g. anencephaly, open spina bifida
- Oesophageal and duodenal atresia

- In many other foetal abnormalities
- Foetal death

4. Chromosomal Abnormalities

In high-risk women, amniotic fluid is aspirated between 15 and 18 weeks of gestation when sufficient foetal cells are likely to be recovered. After centrifugation the cellular fraction is cultured. Karyotyping reveals the chromosomal abnormalities like Trisomy-21, 18, 13 as well as sex chromosomal abnormalities. High-risk women in this category are:

- Age more than 35 years
- H/o previous birth of malformed foetus
- Chromosomal abnormality in either of the parents
- Evidence of Down's syndrome or other chromosomal abnormality in the family
- Previous child with neural tube defect.

5. Antenatal Foetal Sex Determination

Foetal sex determination in families with serious X-linked hereditary disorders can be done by:

- Demonstrating nuclear sex chromatin
- Y-chromosome staining
- Cell culture and karyotyping.

Therapeutic Amniocentesis

Hydramnios

This procedure is used to relieve the distressing symptoms of uterine overdistention like difficulty in sleeping, breathing, etc. About 500 ml of the liquor is drained at a time. Repeated removal may be required, asepsis is important.

Time for Procedure

Usually after 14–16 weeks of gestation when the sac is easily accessible and the quantity of the liquor is sufficient.

Anaesthesia

Local infiltration–lignocaine 1%

Instruments

Long lumbar puncture needle no. 20 G, syringe.

Procedure

1. Urinary bladder is emptied by voiding urine.
2. The procedure is carried out preferably under the ultrasonic guidance so as to localize the placenta and avoid its puncturing.
3. A site for puncture is selected below the fundus and lateral to the midline, preferably on the opposite side of the foetal back. Local anesthesia is infiltrated at the site.
4. Lumbar puncture needle is introduced into the amniotic sac and required quantity of amniotic fluid is aspirated.

For diagnostic purposes, usually 10–20 ml of liquor is removed.

The fluid is centrifuged and the cell free supernatant is used for biochemical studies while the cell rich portion is used for foetal cellular study, enzyme studies or for the cell culture.

The cells are cultured for cytogenetic studies.

Risks

- Trauma to the foetus, placenta or umbilical cord
- Infection
- Abortion/preterm labour
- Foetomaternal haemorrhage resulting in sensitization of Rh negative mother carrying Rh positive foetus.

Triple Screen or Multiple Marker Screen Test

Biochemical screening by triple screen test combining other parameters like age and nuchal translucency measured by ultrasonography is currently recommended for screening for Down syndrome, which should precede the amniocentesis.

Low maternal serum alfa fetoprotein (AFP), high β-HCG, low serum estriol along with maternal age specific risk calculation is currently used as screening test for Down syndrome. The test is performed in early second trimester (15–

20 weeks), risk threshold around 1:250 indicates further evaluation on amniotic fluid for fetal karyotype. The test has false positive and false negative results indicating need for expert consultation for decision-making.

Quadruple test consisting of serum AFP, HCG, unconjugated estriol and inhibin A is performed around 15–20 weeks.

USG measurement of Nuchal fold thickness of 6 mm or more increases the diagnostic accuracy. Long bone measurement, nasal bone absence, sandal gap are other parameters considered.

Screening for Down syndrome in first trimester (11–13 weeks) includes, maternal serum free β-HCG, pregnancy associated plasma protein A (PAPP-A), nuchal translucency (NT)–echolucent area seen in longitudinal views of the back of the neck. NT measurement gives inconsistent results unless performed by specially trained sonologists. Screen positive cases can have chorion villus biopsy for confirmation of abnormality following which a safe early termination is possible.

Screening efficacy is improved with both first and second trimester tests combined. Fetal karyotype is offered if either test positive.

Although the risk of baby with Down's increases beyond age 35, around 80% of affected babies are born to women aged less than 35 years. Hence, routine screening is recommended for all pregnancies.

CHORION VILLUS BIOPSY

Biopsy or sampling of the chorionic tissue can be done either transvaginally or transabdominally. It can be an alternative to amniocentesis and can be performed in first trimester (9–11 weeks).

Foetal cells are obtained earlier. Lengthy culture procedures are unnecessary since chorion cells multiply rapidly. Thus, a diagnosis is made earlier and pregnancy can be terminated early for major foetal chromosomal abnormalities.

Procedure related foetal loss is around 2%. Complication rate depends upon the experience of obstetrician.

CORDOCENTESIS (FOETAL BLOOD SAMPLING)

Percutaneous umbilical blood sampling can be performed under ultrasound guidance.

Indications

- *Erythroblastosis foetalis:* To evaluate haemoglobin concentration of the affected foetus for foetal blood transfusion
- Diagnosis of foetal infection–TORCH
- Rapid karyotyping for foetal chromosomal number Diagnosis of foetal genetic disorders: e.g. β-thalassaemia, Duschenne's muscular dystrophy, sickle cell disease, etc.
- Diagnosis and treatment of foetal hypoxia in IUGR babies.

Procedure

- Spinal needle with stylet is introduced under local anaesthesia with full aseptic precautions; under ultrasonic guidance.
- The site of insertion of umbilical cord into placenta is identified. The cord is punctured 1–2 cm from its insertion into the placenta.
- The stylet is removed and foetal blood is aspirated.

Risks

Foetal loss around 1.6%, abortion rate <1%

FOETOSCOPY

Fetoscope is a thin fiberoptic endoscope of 1 mm diameter. Fetoscopy is an endoscopic procedure during pregnancy to visualize the foetus, to obtain foetal tissue samples or to perform fetal surgery. Certain birth defects can complicate labour and lead to significant foetal deformity or death. Foetal surgical techniques utilizing foetal endoscope help the early intervention of such defects to avoid further serious effects.

Therapeutic Scope of Foetoscopy

- Congenital diaphragmatic hernia
- Myelomeningocoele or Spina bifida

- Urinary tract obstruction which if not treated in time will lead to oligohydramnios and pulmonary hypoplasia
- Congenital cystic adenomatoid malformation of lung
- Sacrococcygeal teratoma
- Twin/twin transfusion syndrome
- Acardiac twin

There are two routes of uterine entry for foetoscope

- *Transabdominal:* Performed after 18 weeks of gestation. A small abdominal incision is taken for the foetoscope insertion (Fig. 14.1).
- *Transcervical:* This can be performed in first trimester of pregnancy.

Anaesthesia

Local, regional or general.

Risks

- The risk of foetal loss is about 3–5%.
- Infection in the foetus and/or mother

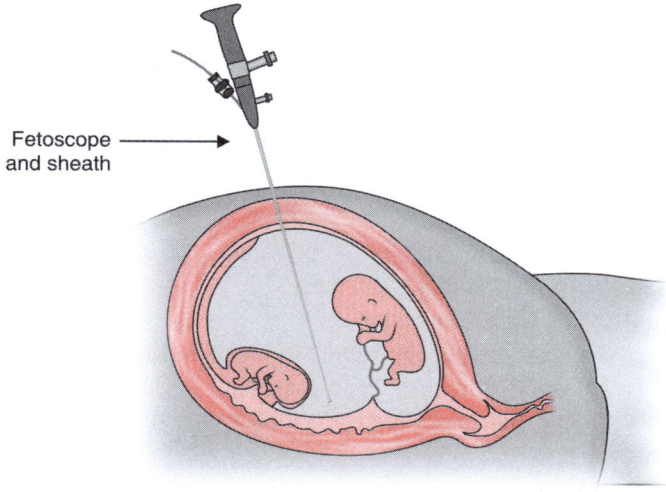

Fetoscope and sheath

Fig. 14.1: Fetoscope

- Premature rupture of amniotic membranes
- Preterm labour

FOETAL TISSUE BIOPSY

Some conditions cannot be diagnosed by any specific molecular genetic test. Prenatal diagnosis of certain conditions can be sometimes accomplished by direct study on foetal tissue. Such tissue is obtained by foetal tissue biopsy performed under ultrasonographic guidance. Following are few examples:
- Muscle biopsy to diagnose muscular dystrophy or mitochondrial myopathy
- Skin biopsy to diagnose epidermolysis bullosa.

The Preconception and Prenatal Diagnostic Techniques (Prohibition of Sex Selection) Act 2003

To prevent the misuse of these techniques in determining the foetal sex and then opting for the sex specific abortions, the Prenatal Diagnostic Techniques Act 1994 has been enforced which has been amended in 2003. The aims of this act are mainly:
- Prevent the misuse of prenatal diagnostic techniques for detection of foetal sex; and thus preventing female foeticide, i.e. female specific abortions.
- Prevent preconceptional sex selection and thus prevent the selection of only male child
- Thus check the diminishing female to male ratio in the society.

The provisions of the amended Act include
- Classification of the genetic centers
- Registration of genetic centers
- Intimation of USG machines
- Authorization of the medical specialists to perform the techniques
- Specifying the penalties for the violation of the Act.

Genetic Centers
- Genetic counseling centre

- *Genetic clinic:* Place which is used for conducting prenatal diagnostic procedures.
- *Genetic laboratory:* Where facilities are provided for conducting analysis or tests of samples received from genetic clinic for prenatal diagnostic tests
- *Ultrasonographic center* can be either genetic clinic or genetic laboratory.

Registration of Genetic Centers

All these centers need to be registered with the appropriate Authority. Additional Director of Health, Family Welfare, MCH and School Health is State Appropriate Authority. On his behalf, Civil Surgeon Acts as Appropriate Authority at District level while Medical Officer of Health carries this responsibility in the area under Municipal Corporation. The Superintendents of Rural Hospitals are Sub-appropriate Authorities. The other Appropriate Authorities are Additional Collectors, Sub-divisional Officers, Tahsildars, Nayab Tahasildars, Commissioners, Deputy Commissioners and Ward Officers of Municipal Corporation and Chief Officers of Municipal Councils.

The registration is to be done with appropriate authority by applying on form A with inclusion of the stipulated Registration Fees (Rs 25000 for any one service and Rs 35000 for centers providing combination of services or institutions). Failure to register the center is an offense for which the equipment can be sealed and seized.

On registration, a certificate of registration is issued which needs to be displayed prominently in the centre. The registration is valid for five years and needs renewal by reapplying and payment for the fees, which is 50% of that required for fresh registration.

Any change in place, employees or equipment has to be intimated to the appropriate authority in writing within thirty days.

The staff appointed at these centers need to be appropriately qualified.

The tests are to be performed only by the authorized persons such as gynecologist, imaging specialists/sonologist as specified in the rules framed by the government.

The manufacturer is to inform the government of sale of every USG machine. The purchaser has to submit an affidavit that he/she will not conduct sex determination of foetus. Ultrasound machine and other equipment capable of detecting fetal sex will be sold only to registered genetic centers.

The procedures can be performed only for conditions specified in the Rules.

Written consent of pregnant woman to undergo the procedure explaining the side effects and after effects of such procedures is necessary. The consent is to be obtained in duplicate in Form G if any invasive procedure is to be performed. A copy of it is to be handed over to the concerned pregnant woman and the other copy is retained in the centre.

Determination of fetal sex is prohibited and communicating fetal sex to any person by words, signs or in any other manner is prohibited.

A copy of the Act should be kept at the centre. The centre should display the information that it does not perform any sex determination.

Authorization of the Medical Specialists

Gynaecologist (having postgraduate qualification in the subject of Gynaecology) is authorized to perform prenatal diagnostic procedures like chorion villus biopsy, amniocentesis, foetoscopy, any foetal organ biopsy or foetal blood sampling. Any registered medical practitioner having experience of carrying out such 20 procedures under supervision of a Gynaecologist is also authorized to perform such prenatal diagnostic procedures.

Radiologist or **imaging scientist** (having postgraduate qualification in Radiology or Ultrasonology or Imageology) is authorized to perform ultrasonography. Any registered medical practitioner having postgraduate degree or six months training or one year experience in sonography or image scanning in a training institute recognized by medical council of India, is also authorized to conduct ultrasonography. He can visit maximum two ultrasonography centres.

Prenatal Diagnostic Procedures

- Ultrasonography
- Fetoscopy
- Chorion villus biopsy
- Amniocentesis
- Cordocentesis
- Foetal biopsy

These procedures may be performed for diagnosis of:
- Chromosomal abnormalities
- Genetic metabolic disorders
- Haemoglobinopathies
- Sex linked genetic diseases
- Congenital anomalies
- Definitely not for the sake of foetal sex detection for sex specific abortions.

Offences and Penalties

Every offence under this Act is cognizable, non-bailable and non-compoundable.

Determining fetal sex, performing the procedures at a place which is not registered for the purpose or by unauthorized persons, communicating fetal sex in any manner, advertising sex selection or sex determination facility in any manner, failure to maintain the required records constitute offenses under this Act and are punishable.

For the first incidence of violation of the Act, the penalties are, fine up to Rs. 10000 and imprisonment up to 3 years. For subsequent offence, these are, fine up to Rs. 50000 and imprisonment up to 5 years.

The appropriate authority can report the name of such medical practitioner to state medical council for removal of name for a period of 5 years for first offence and permanently for subsequent offence(s).

Any person (e.g. family member) seeking aid of a center or a specialist for conducting prenatal diagnosis for purposes other than those specified in the Act or for sex selection is liable for imprisonment up to 3 years and fine up to 50000 rupees for first offence and imprisonment up to 5 years and fine up to 1,00,000 rupees for subsequent offence(s). This does not apply for woman who was pressurized to undergo these tests.

Record Maintenance

All centers have to maintain proper registers and case records which may be inspected by the appropriate authority. Records should be preserved for 2 years; if the legal procedure is on, then the documents should be preserved till the case is dismissed by the court. Appropriate authority has the power to search and seize the records.

The record maintenance is to be done in the specific prescribed forms. Each type of the genetic centre has to maintain their records in different type of forms:

- Genetic counseling centre   Form D
- Genetic laboratory   Form E
- Genetic clinic   Form F
- Informed consent   Form G
  (only for invasive procedures)

Referral letter, declaration by the doctor, signed informed consent form of patient stating that the test is not being done for sex determination are to be maintained.

15

Version

These are manipulative procedures to correct the abnormal foetal presentation.

Types
- External cephalic version
- Internal podalic version

EXTERNAL CEPHALIC VERSION

Abnormal presentation is corrected per abdominally so that the foetus presents by its head.

Indications

Breech presentation or transverse/oblique lie at 36 weeks, as after this point the likelihood of spontaneous version is low.

Why not before 34 weeks?
- Till 34 weeks of pregnancy, due to small size of the foetus and more liquor, the foetus is continuously changing its position. Abnormal presentation before this period therefore, does not carry any significance.
- Spontaneous reversion is more likely
- If patient goes in labour after version, the chances of survival of the newborn are better after 34 weeks than before.

Contraindications

When vaginal delivery is contraindicated (placenta previa, nonassuring fetal status) or when other risk indicators are present:

- Contracted pelvis
- Antepartum haemorrhage
- Previous caesarean section
- Severe hypertension
- Elderly primigravida
- Bad obstetric history

Procedure

- Can be performed in out patient department.
- Prior ultrasonography to rule out fetal anomalies, for adequacy of amniotic fluid volume and to identify placental location.
- For Rh –ve women anti D gamma globulin if indicated.

No anesthesia or premedication is required.

Patient should be in dorsal position with her legs slightly flexed. Obstetrician stands on the right side of the patient.

1. Foetal position is palpated carefully and foetal heart auscultated.
2. Breech is grasped by right hand and displaced from the pelvic brim.
3. Head is grasped with the other hand and pushed towards the flanks in the direction that would increase the flexion.
4. The hands should be changed to complete the version when the foetus assumes transverse position.

Caution

a. The procedure is carried out with utmost gentleness.
b. After completion of the procedure
   - Watch for bleeding or leaking per vaginum.
   - Auscultate foetal heart. If bradycardia persists for more than half an hour, then the version has to be undone. Perform NST if available.
   - Watch for painful uterine contractions; in which case tocolytic agents should be administered.

Complications

- Failed version
- Premature uterine contractions
- Premature separation of placenta
- Accidental rupture of membranes
- Foetal bradycardia
- Rarely, true knot of the cord which causes foetal distress in second stage of labour
- If undue force is applied during the procedure; there is remote possibility of uterine rupture.

Follow-up

After version, the patient is reexamined after a period of one week to confirm whether the corrected lie is maintained. If again the foetus has attained its original position, then external cephalic version may be tried once again. As the foetus grows in size and liquor diminishes, the lie gets stabilized.

Success rate around 60–65%.

Success More Likely

- Muliparity
- Adequate amniotic fluid
- Unengaged presenting part
- Relaxed uterus

Failed Version Likely

- Primigravida with tight abdominal muscles
- Oligohydramnios
- Obese patient
- Very apprehensive patient
- Irritable uterus
- Presenting part engaged
- Frank breech
- Anterior placenta
- Undiagnosed multiple pregnancy/foetal abnormality : This should not occur as USG is usually done before.

Action

1. Ultrasonography to:
   - Exclude major foetal anomaly like anencephaly, hydrocephaly
   - Confirm the type of the breech
   - Exclude multiple pregnancy
2. Hospitalise the patient to attempt version next day after a good night sleep in head low position if no adverse finding is detected.
3. Tocolytics, intravenous ritodrine infusion or subcutaneous turbutaline may improve success.
4. If version fails or is contraindicated, assess the patient fully to decide the safe route of delivery–vaginal or abdominal.

Place of ECV

Successful correction of breech reduces vaginal breech deliveries and caesarean deliveries for breech.

INTERNAL PODALIC VERSION

In this procedure the foetal presentation is changed to breech by intrauterine manipulations.

Formerly this procedure was widely practised for variety of indications in prolonged obstructed labour. However, in modern obstetrics it has got very limited scope, due to its serious complications.

Indications

1. Transverse lie of the second foetus in twin pregnancy.
2. Selected cases of transeverse lie:
   - Multiparous patient
   - Cervix fully or almost fully dilated
   - Membranes intact or recently ruptured with sufficient amount of liquor in uterine cavity.
   - Uterus contracting and relaxing well between the contractions.
   - Average sized baby
   - Adequate pelvis

Anaesthesia

Deep general anaesthesia by ether or halothane to relax the uterus.

Procedure

1. Patient is given lithotomy position, painted and draped.
2. The bladder is catheterised.
3. A gloved whole hand is introduced inside the uterine cavity to reach the breech. From there, one of the lower extremities is traced along the thigh to reach foot and the foot is grasped. The foot is identified and differentiated from hand by feeling the heel. The foot, which is encountered first, should be grasped and brought down. However, if possible, an attempt should be made to bring down the anterior leg first; as anterior buttock may get arrested on the symphysis pubis if posterior leg is pulled down first, resulting in delay in the delivery of the foetus.
4. Simultaneously head of the foetus is pushed up per abdominally by the other hand.
5. Usually internal podalic version is followed by breech extraction for delivering the foetus immediately.
6. Uterine cavity should be explored after delivering the baby for any rent in the uterus.

Complications

- High foetal mortality due to:
  a. Stress of version
  b. Risk of breech delivery is increased by rapid breech extraction
- Uterine rupture

16 Episiotomy

Episiotomy is a deliberate incision made on perineum for easy delivery of the foetus by enlarging the introitus.

Purpose
- Prevent irregular perineal tears
- Effect easy delivery
- Cut short the second stage of labour
- Protect the foetal head from compression and intracranial haemorrhage due to tentoreal tears.

Indications
1. Primigravidae
2. Rigid perineum, irrespective of parity
3. Breech delivery—to shorten the time for the delivery of the after coming head and thus minimising the period of cord compression
4. Instrumental delivery
5. Premature baby—to protect the soft foetal head from compression during delivery and to prevent intracranial haemorrhage
6. Prolonged second stage
7. To cut short the second stage of labour in maternal diseases like heart disease, severe preeclampsia, where maternal bearing down needs to be avoided.

Routine episiotomy may increase the risk of vertical transmission of HIV in HIV infected mother hence avoided.

Anaesthesia

Local perineal infiltration to block the perineal branches of posterior cutaneous femoral nerve and dorsal cutaneous branches of pudendal nerve is usually preferred.

Timing

- At the crowning of head
- Buttocks distending the perineum
- Before or after introduction of the forceps blades.

Types

- Median
- Mediolateral–commonly practised for its advantages (Table 16.1)
- J-shaped
- Lateral

Layers Incised in Episiotomy

Skin, urogential septum, muscles and vagina.

Muscles Incised

- Superficial and deep transverse perineal muscles
- Bulbospongiosus
- Few of the anterior fibres of puborectalis portions of levator ani

Table 16.1: Mediolateral vs median episiotomy	
Mediolateral	*Median*
• Does not lead to third degree perineal tear even if it extends	• Risk of third degree perineal tear if it extends accidently
• More bleeding and pain	• Bleeding and pain minimum
• Incision can be extended, if required	• Limitations to extension due to proximity to anus
• Requires skilled approximation	• Easy to approximate

Suturing

Episiotomy is sutured immediately after the delivery.

Posterior vaginal wall is sutured by continuous sutures with chromic catgut no. 3/0 on atraumatic curved needle. The suturing is started from the apex of the vaginal cut. The mucocutaneous junctions on both the edges are approximated by proper alignment. The muscles are sutured by interrupted sutures and the skin is approximated by interrupted sutures.

Precautions

- Complete haemostasis should be achieved.
- No dead space should be left while suturing the muscles to avoid haematoma formation.

Immediate Complications

a. *Haematoma:* Vulvar, paravaginal or ischiorectal, resulting in swelling and pain
b. Infection and non-union of wound.

Delayed Complications

a. Fibrosis and dyspareunia
b. Implantation dermoid
c. Scar endometriosis

Postoperative Care

1. *Perineal care:*
    - Cleaning the wound after each bowel and bladder action: Cleaning should be done from before backwards in a single stroke action to prevent anal contamination
    - Application of antiseptic cream
    - Use of sterile pads which are frequently changed
    - Inspection of the wound periodically for redness, purulent discharge or any other sign of infection.
2. Removal of perineal skin stitches after five days (if nonabsorbable or when indicated).

Routine vs Selective Episiotomy

Routine use of episiotomy has been shown to be having more posterior perineal trauma (anal sphincter and rectal tears) and other complications as compared to restricted use, hence it should be used selectively when indicated.

It does not prevent the pelvic relaxation as was thought earlier.

PERINEAL TEARS (IRREGULAR LACERATIONS OF PERINEUM)
Etiology

- Precipitate labour
- Unattended labour
- Mismanaged second stage–perineum not supported
- Instrumental delivery, e.g. forceps
- Delivery of a large foetus
- Breech, face, face to pubes delivery
- Rigid perineum
- Delivery through a narrow pubic arch
- Delivery of a primigravida.

Prevention

- Careful conduct of the second stage of labour
- Timely and adequate episiotomy.

Degrees

- *First:* Lacerations of perineal skin/vaginal mucosa.
- *Second:* First degree tear with lacerations of the perineal muscles; but anal sphincter not injured.
- *Third:* Anal sphincter and/or anal mucosa also injured.

Magagement

A. *First and Second Degree Perineal Tears*

- Repair should be done soon after delivery.
- Method of repair and postoperative perineal care is similar to that of episiotomy.

B. *Third Degree Tear*

- Repair has to be done with utmost care in operation theatre and preferably under general anaesthesia.
- Anal mucosa is sutured with 3/0 chromic catgut on atraumatic needle by interrupted sutures. The knots of these sutures are kept inside the lumen of the anal canal. However, suturing of the bowel mucosa may be avoided.
- Suture the muscle wall of the rectum and anal canal by interrupted catgut sutures.
- The retracted ends of the anal sphincters should be identified, grasped with Allis forceps and are approximated with two or three fine catgut sutures.
- The vagina is separated from the rectum for at least 1 cm above the apex of the tear and then suturing is started from the apex. This avoids leaving a gap resulting into a small rectovaginal fistula.

Postoperative Care

- Low residue diet
- Less ambulation
- No enema
- Antibiotics
- Liquid paraffin twice daily.

Complications

1. Wound infection
2. Repair may break requiring delayed repair
3. Incompletely repaired tears may result into rectovaginal fistula.

Subsequent Labour

After Repair of Third Degree Perineal Tear

If easy delivery is anticipated, then it should be conducted with a generous episiotomy. If previous repair had been very difficult or if there is any anticipated delay in labour, caesarean section is preferred.

17

Instrumental Vaginal Delivery

The term instrumental vaginal delivery includes obstetrics forceps and vacuum extractor, which are used to hasten the completion of second stage of labour.

OBSTETRIC FORCEPS

Obstetric forceps were first invented by Peter Chamberlene in sixteenth century. Since then they have undergone number of modifications and improvements. Obstetric forceps are classified as:

1. *Classic instruments*
   - *Long forceps:* Simpson's forceps (Fig. 17.1)
   - *Short forceps:* Wrigley forceps, Simpson's forceps (Fig. 17.2)

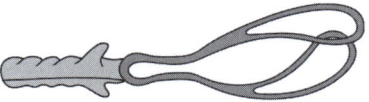

Fig. 17.1: Long forceps

2. *Specialized instruments*
   - Kjelland's forceps
   - Moolgaokar forceps
   - Hay's forceps

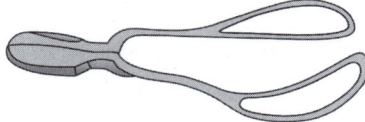

Fig. 17.2: Short forceps

Parts of Obstetric Forceps

Consist of a pair of blades with following parts:

- Handle
- Shank
- *Lock:* Three types—English, Sliding, French
  - *English lock:* This is a common method of articulation of the blades. It consists of a socket located on the shank at its junction with the handle, into which fits a socket situated on the opposite shank.
  - *Sliding lock:* This type of lock is used in Kjelland's forceps in which a single U-shaped receptacle mounted midway on the left shank accepts the shank of the right blade. This type of lock helps correction of asynclitism due to its sliding mechanism.
  - *French lock:* This lock comprises of threaded eye bolt screwed partway into a threaded hole in the left shank and notch in the right shank that articulates with the eye bolt.
- *Fenestrated blade:* They have two curves, pelvic curve to negotiate the pelvis and cephalic curve to accommodate the head of the foetus.

Levels of Forceps

ACOG has classified the forceps delivery with reference to the station and rotation of the head. Three major subdivisions of forceps have been defined (Table 17.1):

- Outlet forceps
- Low forceps
- Midforceps

Types of Application of Blades

Cephalic: The blades are applied along the sides of the foetal head in a line running from the point of chin to the point on vertex near the posterior fontanelle. This is safe procedure.

Pelvic: The blades of the forceps are applied in relation to the pelvic walls irrespective of the position of the foetal head. If

Table 17.1: Based on American Academy of pediatrics and the American College of Obstetricians and Gynecologists (2002)

Type of procedure	Classification
• Outlet forceps	• The foetal head is at or on the perineum • Scalp is visible at the introitus without separating the labia • Foetal skull has reached the pelvic floor • Sagital suture is in anteroposterior diameter or right or left occiput anterior or posterior position • Rotation does not exceed 45°
• Low forceps	• Leading point of foetal skull is at or below station + 2 cm, and not on pelvic floor • Rotation <= 45° • Rotation >45°
• Midforceps	• Station above + 2 cm but head is engaged
• High forceps	• Not included in classification

the foetal head is unrotated, this type of application can cause serious compression of the skull.

When the head is fully rotated the cephalic and pelvic applications coincide with each other (Table 17.2).

Actions of Forceps

• Traction
• Stimulating uterine contractions
• Compression of foetal head to some extent
• Rotation of the head (Kjelland's forceps or Scanzoni's manoeuvre)
• To provide a protective cage for the head.

Table 17.2: Standard measurements		
Measurement	Simpson's long forceps	Wrigley's short forceps
• Distance between the tips	2.50 cm	2.50 cm
• Widest distance between blades	7.50 cm	7.50 cm
• Length of forceps	37.00 cm	27.50 cm
• Radius of cephalic curve	11.25 cm	
• Radius of pelvic curve	17.50 cm	

Indications

1. Prolonged second stage of labour: When second stage duration exceeds 2 hours in primi and 1 hour in multi without any apparent major obstruction.
2. Rigid perineum: Undue resistance to the delivery by maternal soft tissues.
3. Foetal distress in second stage, cord prolapse in second stage
4. Maternal exhaustion in second stage
5. Prophylactic: To cut short the second stage of labour
   - Maternal conditions like heart disease, pre-eclampsia, eclampsia, post-caesarean labour, severe anaemia, diabetes mellitus, etc.
   - Preterm delivery: To give protection to the foetal head from the intracranial haemorrhage. However, not proved to be beneficial for small fetus.
   - Post maturity
6. Aftercoming head in breech to avoid undue delay
7. Occipitosacral (face to pubes) delivery
8. Rotation with traction: Deep transverse arrest–Kjelland's forceps or Scanzoni's manoeuvre.

Criteria to be Fulfilled before Application of Forceps

- Presentation must be suitable and correctly known.
- Head must be engaged deeply and should not be palpable abdominally.
- Cervix must be fully dilated.
- There should be no cephalopelvic disproportion and the pelvic outlet must be adequate.
- Uterus must be contracting; and relaxing between contractions.
- Urinary bladder must be empty.
- Membranes must be ruptured.
- Episiotomy must be given.
- There must be a genuine indication to shorten the second stage.
- Position of vertex must be correctly known.

- For safety, preferably the head should be fully flexed (posterior fontanelle felt easily) and fully rotated (sagittal suture in anteroposterior diameter of the outlet).

Anaesthesia

Usually forceps application is performed under pudendal block. Pre- or intraoperative sedative is not advised for fear or foetal depression. If patient is already under epidural analgesia, then forceps can be applied under the same.

Pudendal Block

A skin wheal is raised by 1% lignocaine half way between the anus and the ischial tuberosity. With index finger in the vagina, ischial spine is palpated and long needle inserted through the wheal is guided to the ischial spine. Then the needle is further pushed just below and behind the ischial spine. At this point, 10 ml of lignocaine is injected. This blocks the internal pundendal nerve just before it enters Alcock's canal. The needle is then withdrawn to the skin level and pushed after changing its direction laterally towards ischial tuberosity. In this region, 5 ml of the anaesthetic agent is infiltrated which blocks perineal branches of posterior cutaneous femoral nerve. The remaining nerves are blocked by guiding the needle from the point of the wheal subcutaneously to the points lateral to the vulva to avoid the pain arising due to the stretching of the introitus during extraction of the head by forceps.

Pundendal block can be given by transvaginal approach also. But due to presence of head in the vagina, usually it is not preferred.

After successful pundendal block, the anus gapes.

Application of the Forceps

1. Patient is given lithotomy position.
2. Parts are painted and draped.
3. Bladder is emptied by catheter.
4. Pudendal block is given.
5. Episiotomy is given at this stage or after introducing the blades.

6. *Introduction of blades:* The left and right blades are indentified. Left blade is introduced first. Left blade is held in the left hand vertically and index and middle fingers of right hand are introduced in the vagina posteriorly. Then the left blade is introduced posteriorly over the two fingers of the right hand. The blade is then swiped in a long arc under the guidance of the fingers laterally. The handle of the blade is depressed over the forchette and the assistant is asked to hold it in position. Then the right blade is introduced in the same way. Correctness of the application is checked.

7. *Locking of the blades:* Correctly applied blades lock very easily without any difficulty.

8. *Traction:* Traction should be given only during uterine contractions. In between the contractions, no traction should be applied, the lock should be disengaged and the pressure on the head of the foetus should be released.

   - Only minimum force should be used during traction. Traction exerted by unaided efforts of the forearm should be adequate and safe. If considerable force becomes necessary, then complete review of the case is advisable.
   - The direction of the traction should be downwards and backwards initially (to maintain the flexion of the head), then in straight direction and finally in the forward direction at the time of delivery of the head.
   - Traction should not be sustained for more than 8 to 10 seconds and each series of three to four pulls should be followed by clear rest interval to allow the circulation of blood in the foetal brain to be restored.

9. Immediately after the delivery of the head, the blades should be removed.

Criteria for the Correct Application of Blades

1. Good grasp is obtained if the blades are applied correctly.
2. Blades lock readily. If the handles are widely separated, the blades should be removed, careful vaginal examination should be performed to ascertain the position and attitude of the head before reapplication. In such circumstances,

usually the head is found in occipitolateral or occipito-posterior position.

3. Position of lambdoidal suture is a good guide to judge the correctness of the application of the forceps blades. The distance between the lambdoidal suture and the anterior edge of each forceps blade is small—about 2 cm and is same on both sides.
4. The sagittal suture should bisect the space between the forceps blades posteriorly (Fig. 17.3).
5. The operator should be unable to accomodate more than a finger tip between the fenestration of the blade and the foetal head on either side.

Complications

Maternal

Immediate

1. Perineal tears–even third degree tear may occur
2. Vaginal lacerations
3. *Cervical tears:* If the forceps application is done before full dilatation of the cervix
4. *Traumatic PPH due to tissue injury:* Therefore, it is very important to explore cervix and vagina after forceps delivery.

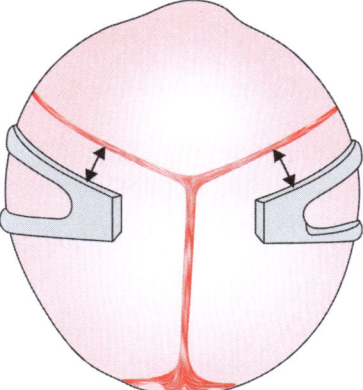

Fig. 17.3: Correct application

5. Cervical tears may extend into the lower uterine segment.
6. Neurogenic shock
7. Injury to urinary bladder leading to vesicovaginal fistula
   • Direct injury
   • Pressure necrosis
8. Injury to nerve trunks of sacral plexus
9. Dislocation of sacroiliac joint

Delayed
10. Genital prolapse

Neonatal

Immediate
• Injury to the face, eyes, facial palsy
• Fracture skull
• Intracranial haemorrhage–undue compression in brow-mastoid application may be dangerous
• Cephalhaematoma
• Asphyxia

Delayed
Birth trauma can lead to neurological complications in later life.

Safe Forceps
• Outlet and low
• Correct cephalic application
• Midforceps to be applied only in carefully selected patients, in operation theatre, by experienced person.

Difficulties in Forceps Delivery
1. Difficulty in introduction of blades
   • Cervix not fully dilated
   • Rotation of head incomplete
2. Difficulty in locking the blades
   • Blades not pushed enough inside vagina
   • Handles not depressed against the perineum
   • Occipitotransverse or occipitoposterior position
   • Deflexed head

3. Difficulty in traction
   • Selection of unsuitable case
   • Improper application of blades–not cephalic
   • Persistent occipitoposterior position or brow presentation
   • Traction in wrong direction
   • Occasional case of outlet contraction
4. Slipping of blades
   • Persistent occipitoposterior position
   • Hydrocephalus

TRIAL FORCEPS

A tentative application of forceps with anticipated difficulty in delivering the patient with forceps is called as *Trial Forceps*.

Since failure to effect delivery after trial forceps demands caesarean section and that too without wasting much time; in the interest of the foetus, it has to be carried out only in well equipped operation theatre with preparations for caesarean section ready.

FAILED FORCEPS

Failure to deliver the patient with forceps is called as *Failed Forceps*. In such condition the case is to be reviewed properly again. Such cases usually have to be delivered by caesarean section.

Causes

• Undiagnosed cephalopelvic disproportion
• Incompletely dilated cervix
• Persistent occipitoposterior position or deep transverse arrest
• Deflexed head
• Large head/undiagnosed hydrocephalus

Perinatal mortality is very high following failed forceps. Hence, careful selection of cases for forceps delivery and timely caesarean section is essential in difficult cases.

AXIS-TRACTION

- Pelvic axis is curved
- If the line of traction is not in the line with the pelvic axis, lot of force can go waste against pubic symphysis. Hence, more force is required.
- Axis-traction brings the line of traction in line of pelvic axis; hence less force is required for extraction.

Is Axis-traction Necessary?

The place of axis-traction is when the head is high in the pelvis. Its need goes on diminishing as the head descends down and becomes needless when it reaches the pelvic floor. In modern obstetrics the high forceps application is replaced by caesarean section. In most of the places therefore, axis-traction is replaced by Pajot's manoeuvre.

Pajot's Manoeuvre (Fig. 17.4)

In this manoeuvre, after the application of the forceps, while giving traction, the obstetrician pulls on the handle of the forceps with his right hand, while with his left hand he presses downwards on the shanks. With this manoeuvre, the direction of the force goes on changing as the head starts descending in the pelvic cavity and thus the resistance against the pubic symphysis is avoided.

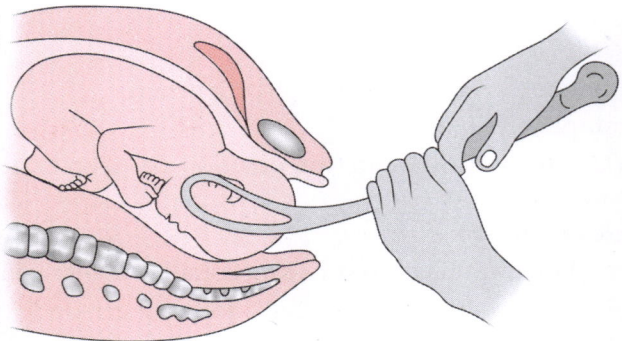

Fig. 17.4: Pajot's manoeuvre

KJELLAND'S FORCEPS (Fig. 17.5)

Indications

- Deep transverse arrest (DTA)
- Persistent occipitoposterior position (POP).

Characteristics

- Long, stout, heavier forceps
- Minimal pelvic curve to enable correct cephalic grip even if the head is arrested in the transverse position.
- Sliding lock to allow a better adjustment of the blades if the head is asynclitic.
- Knobs on the handles to indicate the position of the occiput.

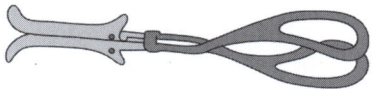

Fig. 17.5: Kjelland's forceps

Action

- Rotation of foetal head
- Traction

Blades

Instead of left and right blades, these blades will be designated as anterior and posterior blades depending upon the position of the foetal head.

1. Confirm the position of the foetal head correctly and decide anterior blade accordingly.
2. There are three methods of introducing anterior blade
   - *Long wandering method:* This is the commonly used and safest of all the methods. First, obstetrician introduces his hand in the vagina posteriorly. Then the anterior blade is introduced in sacral hollow and wandered under the guidance of the obstetrician's hand in the vagina over the face or occiput to bring it under the pubic symphysis.

- *Direct method:* Anterior blade is introduced directly behind the pubic symphysis.
- *Classical method:* The anterior blade is placed into the lower uterine segment anteriorly with curve anteriorly placed. Then it is rotated, handle being rotated in a wide circle. The blade is then fixed on the head anteriorly. This method can lead to trauma to the lower uterine segment which already has become soft and thin due to the obstruction in labour.

3. Posterior blade is introduced directly. It is necessary to give a wide deep episiotomy while applying the Kjelland's forceps.

Extraction of Head

- Sliding lock allows the correction of the asynclitism.
- Traction is given only during the uterine contractions.
- Rotation of the head is done in between the contractions.

Complications

- High incidence of spiral vaginal tears
- Injury to the lower uterine segment

In view of the associated morbidity this forceps is not commonly used.

Precautions

Cephalopelvic disproportion–particularly midpelvic and outlet–often responsible for DTA should be carefully excluded, in which case, caesarean section is always a safer mode of delivery.

VACUUM EXTRACTOR (VENTOUSE)

Principle

Acceleration of the delivery by effecting traction on foetal head with the help of vacuum cup.

Instrument

There are two general designs of vacuum extractor.

- *Soft cup:* Silastic or soft plastic cups. Preferred as these are safer than metal cup.
- *Rigid cup:* Metal cup of Malmstrom and the modification of Bird and others.

Significant scalp injuries, hematomas and hyperbilirubine-mia are more common with metal cup. Soft cups cause less scalp injury but have somewhat higher failure rates than with metal cups.

With soft cup negative pressure can be increased rapidly. Hence, currently the soft cup instruments are used.

There are special cups suitable for application for occipitoposterior positions (Kiwi omnicup).

Sialastic Cup (Fig. 17.6)

- Soft silicon elastomer cup of 65 mm diameter
- Can shape to the foetal head
- Suction is created without delay
- Negative pressure applied only during traction, hence less scalp trauma
- Difficult placement on deflexed head
- Higher failure rate in occipitoposterior position
- Suitable for easy outlet position.

Mityvac

- Disposable plastic cup of 60 mm diameter
- Cup has deeper dome like a tea cup
- No necessity to form Chignon
- Safer than metal cup

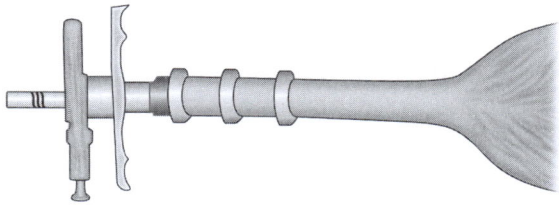

Fig. 17.6: Sialastic cup

Components of Malmstrom Vacuum Extractor

- Cup to fit on the scalp of foetal head having a knob on it for indicating the position of occiput.
- Metal plate inside the cup
- A chain inside the rubber tube. This chain is attached to metal plate at one end and to the pin in the traction bar at the other end.
- Suction bottle with accurate manometer and a valve to the nozzle to which suction pump is connected.
- A rubber tube to connect traction bar to the suction bottle
- Suction pump to create vacuum inside the bottle
- *The cups of three sizes:* 40 mm, 50 mm and 60 mm. The greatest diameter of the cup is at a level of 8 mm from the point of application to the scalp.

Bird's Cup

The traction chain and the vacuum tube are separate. There is a hook in the center of the cup to which traction chain is attached. The vacuum chain is placed eccentrically or at the side of the cup. Thus the problem of detachment during traction is avoided.

Indications

To cut short the second stage of labour. Prerequisites for use are the same as for forceps delivery.

Application and Use

Correct application of cup over the foetal head is the key to the success and safety of vacuum extractor.

1. Cervix must be fully dilated.
2. The vacuum cup is positioned midline over the sagittal suture with its centre lying 6 cm behind bregma; around 3 cm in front of posterior fontanelle. Correct application is confirmed (Fig. 17.7).
3. Vacuum is created and traction is given on the cup.
4. The traction should be synchronous with the uterine contractions, with the maternal expulsive force and at right

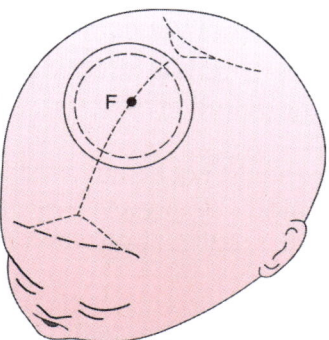

Fig. 17.7: Placement of cup

angle to the cup. The traction should be applied in the direction of the axis of the pelvis. Therefore, the perineum should be depressed by two fingers. For the head in the midcavity, it is advisable to press the margin of the cup by a finger into the sacral hollow.

5. The other hand can be placed within the vagina to:
   • Palpate foetal scalp with one or two fingers
   • Place thumb on the cup to provide counter pressure and for noting the relative position of the cup edge to the scalp.
6. If the cup slips it can be repositioned.
7. Abandon the procedure if
   • Cup slips twice
   • Delivery not effected within four pulls or within 15–20 minutes.

While using Malmstrom's metal cup, a hand pump is used to exhaust the air and create vacuum. Initially, suction just sufficient to fix the cup to the foetal scalp, i.e. up to 0.2 kg/sq. cm is obtained. Full required suction (0.7–0.8 kg/sq cm) to create vacuum is applied to form a good Chignon, which is an artificial caput created inside the cup by means of vacuum. The traction is then exerted on the foetal head through the chain contained within the suction tube attached to the cup.

Check Points for Correct Vacuum Extractor Placement

- Vacuum port or the handle is directed towards foetal head.
- The cup should be placed midsagittal with the edge of cup 3 cm from Bregma.
- Maternal tissue should not be included in the cup.
- Application should be *flexing and median*.
- Deflexing and paramedian application to be avoided.

Advantages

1. Minimal maternal analgesia required
2. Can be applied even if the head is not fully rotated.
3. Can be applied to a deflexed head also.
4. Does not occupy any space in the pelvis.
5. Pulling force is applied to the scalp and not to the base of the skull directly as is applied in forceps. This gives mechanical advantage for traction as long as only moderate traction is applied.
6. With the pull on the vacuum cup, there is autorotation of the head as it descends down. Unlike forceps, it need not be rotated actively.
7. Unlike obstetric forceps, ventouse cannot be abused with a greater force to cause danger, as it will pull off with such a great force.
8. Delivery is more physiological.
9. Incidence of birth trauma to the child is reduced.
10. Risk of maternal injuries is minimal.

Disadvantages

1. Contraindicated in face or breech presentations
2. Unsafe for premature foetus
3. Foetal scalp injuries and serious complications possible
4. Minor skin echimosis and abrasions are possible.
5. Metal cup extraction is a slow process, hence unsuitable in severe foetal distress
6. Chignon gives an ugly appearance to the baby for a few days and may cause maternal apprehension.
7. Use of metal cup as a rotator can result in cookie cutter avulsions of the foetal scalp.

Neonatal Complications

1. Scalp haematoma, sloughing of scalp
2. Cephalohematoma, subgaleal hematoma
3. Intracranial haemorrhage
4. Subconjunctival hemorrhage, retinal hemorrhage
5. Minor skin echimosis and abrasions
6. Hyperbilirubinemia

Contraindications

High station, suspicion of CPD, nonvertex presentation, preterm fetus.

Vacuum extraction carries less maternal complications in comparison to forceps (Table 17.3).

Neither forceps nor vacuum extractor is to be applied at high station or used before full cervical dilatation.

Table 17.3: Forceps vs vacuum extractor

Forceps	Ventouse
• Extraction quick–suitable for distressed foetus	• Extraction slow–unsuitable for distressed foetus
• Safe for preterm foetus	• Unsafe for preterm foetus
• Can be used for face and breech aftercoming head	• Cannot be used in face and breech
• Occupies space in vagina	• Does not occupy space
• Risk of inadvertant use of excessive force	• Excessive force cannot be applied as cup slips
• Risk of genital trauma more	• Minimum risk of genital trauma
• More risk of birth trauma to child	• More neonatal injuries, jaundice
• Complete rotation and flexion of head desirable	• Can be applied to incompletely rotated or deflexed head
• Maternal discomfort more–some anaesthesia required	• Minimum discomfort–no anaesthesia required
• Lithotomy position required– hence unsuitable for cardiac cases	• Can be applied in dorsal position–hence suitable for cardiac cases
• Preferred to vacuum extraction in cases of HIV infected mother	• May cause more microlacerations to foetal scalp and hence possible increased risk of vertical transmission of HIV in HIV infected mother

18 Caesarean Section

Caesarean section is a surgical procedure to deliver a foetus per abdominally through an incision on the uterus.

Historical

This operation though practiced from the period before Julius Caesar, he legalized this procedure, hence the name. In those days, it was customary, not to bury a dead woman in the pregnant state. Following the death of a pregnant woman, her child was being delivered by opening her abdomen before she was buried. If the child also would happen to be dead, a situation often encountered, then the mother and the child were buried separately.

Later on, this procedure was performed on live mothers who could not deliver vaginally. But the maternal mortality in these cases used to be around 70–80% since the uterus was not sutured. This was the state of affairs up to as late as eighth decade of nineteenth century.

Porro of Italy in 1876 introduced a new method of excising the body of the uterus and fixing the cervical stump to the abdominal wound where the bleeding could be controlled by pressure. With this modification, the maternal mortality dropped down to about 35–40%.

In 1881 and 1882, Kehrer and Sanger respectively practiced the suturing of the uterus after caesarean section, though it was first suggested by Lebas in 1769.

Kehrer performed the first Lower Segment Caesarean Section on 25th September, 1881. Before that, the procedure was performed by a vertical incision on the body of the uterus; now known as classical caesarean section.

Types of Caesarean Sections

A. **Lower segment caesarean section:** The uterus is incised on the lower segment by a crescent shaped transverse incision. This is a safe procedure practiced currently. It can be performed as an elective or an emergency procedure (Table 18.1).

B. **Classical caesarean section:** This is the original and the easiest form of caesarean section where the uterus is incised vertically in the midline on the upper segment.

Indications

1. Foetal distress in first stage of labour.
2. Cord prolapse or presentation with live foetus.
3. Cephalopelvic disproportion (CPD)
   - Major degree CPD
   - Minor degree CPD with any other risk factor where trial labour is contraindicated
   - Minor degree CPD where trial labour fails.
4. Previous caesarean section
   - If the indication for previous caesarean section was recurrent one, e.g. contracted pelvis.
   - If previous caesarean section was done after failed trial labour or for prolonged obstructed labour with threatened uterine rupture where integrity of scar is doubtful.
   - Two or more previous caesarean sections
   - Previous classical caesarean section
   - Abnormal presentation, antepartum haemorrhage (APH), severe toxaemia or any other complication in current pregnancy.
5. Malpresentation
   - Transverse lie
   - Brow presentation
   - Mentoposterior face presentation
   - Breech presentation with large baby, doubtful pelvis, hyperextended head or footling breech, preterm breech.

6. Multifetal pregnancy
   - Twins with first baby with transverse lie, noncephalic presentation
   - Second fetus showing nonreassuring FHR patterns
   - Potential for locked twins
   - Triplets or higher order gestation.

7. Prolonged obstructed labour due to:
   - CPD, malpresentations, persistent occipitoposterior position (POP), deep transverse arrest (DTA), etc.
   - *Unsatisfactory progress of labour:* Patient crossing the alert and action line on partograph and unsuitable for oxytocin or not progressing satisfactorily after oxytocin infusion.

8. Placenta praevia
   - Types III, IV, and II posterior
   - Continuous bleeding after amniotomy.

9. Abruptio placentae
   - Concealed hemorrhage with live fetus
   - Failed induction of labour
   - Unsatisfactory progress after induction of labour.

10. Pregnancy induced hypertension (PIH)
   - Fulminating toxaemia where quick termination of pregnancy is necessary for foetal/neonatal safety and the cervix is unripe
   - *Eclampsia:* If the convulsions remain uncontrolled even after 8–10 hours of conservative management and the cervix is unripe.

11. Fetal growth restriction of the foetus with severe foetal jeopardy and cervix unfavorable for induction.

12. Imminent foetal death due to uteroplacental insufficiency as indicated by:
   - Cessation of foetal movements
   - Non-reactive nonstress test with poor variability and spontaneous decelerations
   - Contraction stress test revealing repeated late decelerations

- USG showing poor biophysical profile, liquor volume severely reduced, absence of foetal movements and poor foetal tone.
13. Bad obstetric history (BOH).
14. Elderly primigravidae in association with other abnormalities or pregnancy complications.
15. Some cases of diabetes mellitus, particularly with the history of intrauterine deaths in previous pregnancies or labour.
16. Reduction of the risk of vertical transmission of HIV infection to the baby–prelabour elective caesarean section has been shown to beneficial when the maternal viral load is >1000 copies/ml. However, the benifits have to be weighed against the risk of increased postoperative morbidity.
17. Maternal genital herpes with active genital lesions–to prevent neonatal herpes.
18. Failed induction of labour.
19. Incoordinate uterine action causing foetal distress.
20. Rigid cervix causing cervical dystocia.
21. History of repair operation for urinary or rectal incontinence.
22. History of any surgery on the uterus leaving a vulnerable scar on the uterus.
23. Pelvic tumors causing obstruction.
24. Structural abnormalities of uterus/vagina.
25. Carcinoma cervix diagnosed very late in pregnancy.
26. Carcinoma rectum diagnosed late in pregnancy.

Preoperative

- Exclude/correct anaemia.
- Use of ultrasonography for placental localization, assessment of foetal maturity and exclude foetal malformations
- Informed consent
- Patient should be kept nil by mouth for 8 hours.
- Simple enema
- Abdomen and perineum should be prepared.

- Intravenous infusions for correcting any dehydration or acidosis of the mother during labour
- Catheterize the bladder and retain the catheter throughout the surgery to avoid accidental injury to the bladder.
- Keep all the measures of neonatal resuscitation ready.

Anaesthesia

Caesarean section is performed under spinal, epidural or general anaesthesia. Under certain emergency conditions, the surgery can be performed under local anaesthesia.

Spinal Anaesthesia

Spinal anaesthesia is induced by lignocaine 5% intrathecally.

Advantages
- Quick action
- Operative and postoperative haemorrhage is reduced since the uterine retraction is not interfered with.
- Very little postoperative vomiting hence suitable for the patients who are not on empty stomach
- No effect on baby
- Early reappearance of peristalsis
- Rapid postoperative recovery
- Easy to initiate early breastfeeding
- Effect on kidneys and liver is negligible.

Disadvantages
- Severe hypotension
- Higher blockade possible due to small subarachinoid space
- Spinal headache
- Rarely convulsions
- Bladder dysfunction
- Hypertension more common following Inj. Methergin
- Infection
- Failed block possible (requiring general anesthesia)
- Unsuitable in maternal coagulopathy, mothers receiving heparin injections, suspicion of neurological disease, infection at the injection site.

Table 18.1: Elective vs emergency caesarean section

	Elective	Emergency
1. Decision	Preplanned surgery	Emergency surgery
2. Common indications	• Major degree CPD • Elderly primigravida with other high risk factors • Previous two or more caesarean sections	• Foetal distress • Maternal distress, APH • Failed trial labour
3. Merits and demerits	*Advantages* • Experienced team of surgeons and anaesthetist can be made available • Well prepared patient—empty stomach • Cross-matched blood can be kept ready *Disadvantages* • Risk of birth of preterm baby, hence gestational age should be ascertained correctly • Slightly higher risk of PPH due to uterine atony	*Disadvantages* • Skilled surgeons and anaesthetist may not be available • Patient may not be well prepared • Blood may not be available *Advantages* • No risk of iatrogenic preterm delivery • Usually uterus is contracting, hence less risk of PPH

Epidural

- Injection of local anesthetic in epidural space
- Volume of epidural space is reduced during pregnancy
- *Lumbar epidural:* Repeated doses can be given through an indwelling catheter, block from T10 to S5 dermatomes.

Complications
- Dural puncture may cause total spinal block
- Ineffective analgesia
- Hypotension (crystalloid preload to avoid)
- Convulsions rarely
- Pyrexia
- Postpartum backache

Combined Spinal Epidural Anesthesia

Quick and sustained action.

General Anaesthesia

Induction is done by Thiopental-Na intravenously, supported by succinylcholine for intubation. Induction after painting and draping minimizes the time between administration of the drug and delivery of the baby and reduces transplacental transfer of Thiopental-Na. The arm-placenta time is 4 minutes. The anaesthesia can be maintained by nitrous oxide and oxygen with intermittent fractional succinylcholine. Minimal use of halothane or isoflurane to avoid relaxant action on the uterus to minimize the chances of atonic postpartum haemorrhage.

Disadvantages
- Depression of foetus
- Uterine atony
- Vomiting is more common with increased risk of Mendleson's syndrome due to aspiration of vomitus, therefore unsuitable for patients with full stomach
- Failed intubation more often during pregnancy
- Safety less as compared to regional block.

LOWER SEGMENT CAESAREAN SECTION

A transverse crescent shaped incision is taken in the lower uterine segment through a transperitoneal approach.

Instruments
- General instruments for laparotomy
- Doyen's retractor
- Green-Armytage forceps.

Steps of Operation
1. Patient is given dorsal position and bladder is catheterized.
2. Anterior abdominal wall is opened in layers through transverse abdominal incision (Pfannensteil or Joel Cohen incision). It has less postoperative pain and for its cosmetic effect as compared to subumbilical midline vertical incision
3. After reaching the peritoneal cavity, the uterus is brought in the midline by correcting the dextrorotation if any. Round ligaments help to judge the uterine position.
4. Lower segment is identified by overlying loose peritoneum.
5. Loose peritoneal reflection of the uterovesical pouch is incised above the level of the urinary bladder.
6. The bladder along with the fold of peritoneum is separated from the anterior wall of the lower segment of uterus and pushed low down to the safe level by fingers or swab on holder.
7. The bladder is retracted by Doyen's retractor.
8. A small incision is taken in the anterior wall of the lower segment through its full thickness.
9. The incision is extended laterally on both the sides curving upwards. Blunt expansion is preferred over sharp one.
10. Four fingers of the right hand are inserted between the lower flap of the lower segment and below the leading point on the head of the baby so that the head of the baby rests on the palm of the hand. Doyen's retractor is removed at this stage.

11. Levering with the hand, by maintaining the flexion the head is elevated into the uterine and abdominal incision and is delivered. Then the shoulders are delivered. Finally the trunk is delivered.
12. The cord is clamped and severed.
13. Angles of the uterine incision and the edges are caught by Green-Armytage forceps in order to minimize the bleeding through the edges of the incision.
14. At this stage oxytocic (oxytocin 5 IU) is administered intravenously slowly.
15. Placenta and the membranes are delivered by controlled cord traction.
16. The uterine incision is closed in two layers by chromic catgut or vicryl no. 1 on round body curved needle by continuous interlocking sutures. Safety of single layer closure is uncertain. Intraperitoneal closure is performed without exteriorization of the uterus. Peritoneum of vesico-uterine pouch is generally left unsutured
17. Proper and effective haemostasis is ensured.
18. The abdomen is closed in layers.

Advantages of Lower Segment Caesarean Section

1. The uterine wall of lower segment is thin, particularly in established labour. Hence, accurate approximation of the edges is possible.
2. After delivery, unlike body of the uterus, lower segment is quiescent. Therefore, wound healing is better.
3. The area of scar being less dynamic, there are less chances of rupture in subsequent labour.
4. As the wound is covered by peritoneum the convalescence is smooth, there are less chances of forming adhesions. It is safer in infected cases.
5. The lower segment contains more fibrous tissue than the body of the uterus, hence it is less vascular. Therefore, amount of bleeding during surgery is much less than in classical caesarean section.
6. Complications are less in comparison to classical caesarean.

Dangers and Risks

Immediate

1. Haemorrhage
   - Usually bleeding from the uterine incision is not alarming and easily gets controlled after the uterus is sutured.
   - Opening of uterine vessels by lateral extension of incision may cause alarming bleeding from the angles of the incision. Catching them and suturing controls such bleeding but while doing so care should be taken not to include ureter in the ligature.
   - Uterine atony may cause post-partum haemorrhage. Intravenous administration of ergot preparation and oxytocin controls such bleeding. Intramyometrial or intramuscular injection of 250 µg of 15 methyl PGF2-α controls the bleeding promptly. Uterine massage is also helpful. If these measures fail, conservative surgical procedures are attempted however sometimes hysterectomy may be required to save the life of the patient.
2. Injury to the urinary bladder
3. Trauma to the child
   - By sharp cutting instruments
   - Undue and wrongly directed force while delivering the baby
   - Extraction by breech or shoulder may result in fractures and dislocations.

Late

During postoperative period
1. Paralytic ileus and abdominal distension
2. Infection
   - Wound infection
   - Uterine infection
   - Peritonitis
   - Septicaemia
   - Urinary infection
3. Non-union of wound
4. Secondary postpartum haemorrhage
5. Thromboembolism

Sequelae

1. Incisional hernia
2. Chronic abdominal pain due to adhesions
3. Risk of scar rupture in subsequent pregnancy.

MISGAV LADACH TECHNIQUE

This technique of LSCS has been introduced by Misgav Ladach hospital in Jerusalem.

Steps of Operation

A. *Opening the Abdomen*

- Joel-Cohen incision is given by a superficial cut in the cutis; about 3 cm below an imaginary line between the two anterior-superior iliac spines.
- In the centre, where there are no blood vessels, the cut is made deeper reaching the fascia.
- A small transverse opening is made in the fascia with the tip of a scalpel.
- The fascia is opened transversely underneath the fat tissue and blood vessels by pushing the tip of scissors on either directions.
- The fascia is stretched caudally and cranially by index fingers.
- Now the surgeon and the assistant stretch the muscles, blood vessels and fat by inserting index and middle finger under the muscles and exerting bilateral traction.
- A small hole is created in parietal peritoneum by stretching it by index fingers. This hole is further stretched in caudocranial direction to extend the peritoneal opening transversely.
- Visceral peritoneum is opened
- The bladder is gently pushed down with the index finger.

B. *Opening the Uterus*

- A small midline transverse incision is made in the lower uterine segment until membranes bulge.

- The incision is extended laterally by index finger of one hand and thumb of the other.

C. Delivering the Foetus

- The foetus is delivered as usual.
- Placenta is removed manually.

D. Suturing the Uterus

- Uterus is exteriorised.
- Uterine incision sutured in one layer with locked stitches of chromic catgut no. 1.

E. Closing the Abdomen

- Only large clots if any are removed.
- The uterus is replaced back into abdominal cavity.
- Visceral and parietal peritoneum are not sutured and are left for natural healing.
- The rectus sheath is stitched with continuous nonlocking stitch
- The skin and subcutis are closed with widely spaced silk sutures.

F. Removal of Skin Stitches

Skin stitches are removed on 5th postoperative day.

Advantages

- Operation is short due to rational use of only very essential steps. Unnecessary steps like suturing peritoneum are eliminated.
- Since the tissue separation avoids blood vessels, haemostatic steps and swabbing are not required.
- Incision is placed where the fascia is not attached and moves freely over the muscles. Hence, no need of separating fascia from the muscles.
- Tissues are separated along the connective tissue lines. Therefore, healing is more complete and rapid.
- Reduced febrile morbidity.

- Fewer postoperative adhesions and less pain.
- Short convalescent period and woman can regain herself more rapidly for breastfeeding and care of newborn.

CLASSICAL CAESAREAN SECTION

A vertical incision is taken on the body of the uterus in the midline to open the uterine cavity to deliver the child.

Indications
1. When a large myoma prevents the access to the lower uterine segment.
2. Pregnancy with carcinoma of cervix
3. Extensive adhesions to the abdominal wall by previous surgery preventing the exposure of the lower segment.
4. When multiple previous lower segment caesarean sections have scarred the lower segment to the extent that no room is left for fresh incision and repair.
5. Large and abnormal foetus, e.g. conjoined twins
6. Placenta praevia where
   - The lower segment is extremely vascular.
   - Exsanguinated mother in critical condition.
7. Occasional cases of transverse lie in which identification of the lower segment is not possible
8. Contraction ring dystocia
9. Gross kyphosis
10. *A live baby in dead mother:* Quick delivery of foetus immediately after the death of mother may save the child.

Steps of Operation
1. The abdomen is opened by paramedian incision and the uterus is brought in the centre.
2. An incision of about 10–15 cm in length is taken in the anterior wall of the uterus in the midline, taking care not to encroach beyond the bladder reflection on the lower segment.
3. At this stage, profuse bleeding occurs. Therefore, it is important to deliver the child quickly by catching a leg and giving traction on it.

4. The cord is immediately clamped and severed.
5. The uterus is then partially delivered out of the abdominal cavity through the abdominal incision.
6. The placenta and the membranes are removed.
7. The uterine incision is closed in two layers by series of interrupted sutures by chromic catgut or vicryl no.1 on an atraumatic curved needle.
8. The abdomen is closed in layers.

Advantage
Easy and quick approach is the only advantage.

Disadvantages
- The scar on the uterus is weak and hence more vulnerable for rupture during the subsequent pregnancy and labour.
- The scar is more prone for infections and postoperative period is likely to be stormy.
- Development of intestinal adhesions; sometimes intestinal obstruction may follow classical caesarean section.

Weakness of Classical Scar on Uterus

The scar of classical caesarean section is more vulnerable for rupture during subsequent pregnancy as compared to the lower segment caesarean section scar.

Apart from the fact that the classical scar is in the actively contractile portion of the uterus and hence is more vulnerable for the rupture; it is more important to note that due to the following factors the classical section scar is weak:

1. The wound is more prone to get infected.
2. The uterine muscle fibers are in a state of degeneration in the puerperal period.
3. During the puerperium, the scar region of the uterus is in a state of unrest. The sutures therefore are continuously at stress due to the contractions and relaxations of the uterus; more so in first twenty four hours of puerperium.
4. The midline being less vascular, the healing is impaired.
5. It is virtually impossible to oppose the muscles on the two sides of the scar exactly while suturing the edges as they are

irregularly distributed. This results in the collection of small pockets of blood which in the process of healing are replaced by fibrous tissue in place of the muscle.

6. Invariably, on the endometrial surface, a gutter runs along the scar. During the pregnancy, the membranes herniate through this gutter, further weakening the scar.

7. If the placenta is situated anteriorly, it is difficult to coapt the edges of uterine wound exactly due to its friability with more pronounced tendency to the gutter formation.

8. During subsequent pregnancy, if placenta gets implanted on the scar, the penetrating action of the chorionic villi further weakens the scar.

The comparison of lower segment and classical caesarean sections is shown in Table 18.2. The clinical differences in the scar rupture in subsequent pregnancy following these are shown in Table 18.3.

Subsequent Labour

A common belief *Once a Caesarean, always a Caesarean,* is not true. Vaginal birth after a caesarean (VBAC) section in carefully selected cases helps in reducing the caesarean deliveries.

Whether to allow the next delivery by a vaginal trial or not depends upon following factors:

1. *Indication for the caesarean:* If the indication is recurrent (e.g. contracted pelvis), then the subsequent delivery has to be by caesarean section; but if the caesarean was performed for nonrecurrent indication (e.g. placenta praevia), these cases may be allowed vaginal delivery in future pregnancies.

2. *Type of caesarean section performed:* Women with previous lower segment caesarean may be allowed vaginal deliveries, but once classical caesarean is performed always a caesarean is required.

3. *Number of previous caesarean sections:* Cases with two or more previous caesareans should have a caesarean delivery.

4. *Post caesarean period:* If the post caesarean period was hectic with fever and foul smelling discharge indicating uterine infection, it is very much likely that the scar has remained

Table18.2: Lower segment vs classical caesarean section

Lower segment	Classical
1. Incision on lower segment of uterus usually transverse	1. Uterine incision midline vertical in upper segment
2. Edges of uterine incision thin-easy approximation	2. Edges of uterine incision thick-difficult approximation
3. Technically difficult; need for pushing urinary bladder down	3. Technically easy
4. More time required	4. Quick procedure
5. Better healing of the scar which is situated in the passive lower segment. Hence less chances of scar dehiscence in subsequent pregnancy	5. Scar remains weak being situated in the active contractile portion of the uterus. Hence, chances of scar rupture during subsequent pregnancy considerably high.
6. Uterine wound well covered by uterovesical peritoneum: • Less chances of adhesions • In infected cases less chances of spread of infection to general peritoneal cavity	6. Uterine wound exposed to general peritoneal cavity: • More adhesion formation • More likelihood of spread of infection and general peritonitis in infected cases
7. Postoperative convalescence smooth	7. Chances of stormy postoperative period with abdominal distension requiring prolonged parenteral fluids
8. Vaginal delivery possible in subsequent pregnancy under careful supervision in selected cases	8. Elective caesarean section at 37 weeks obligatory in subsequent pregnancy

Table 18.3: Scar rupture following classical and lower segment caesarean section

Lower segment	Classical
1. Chances about 0.4%	1. Chances about 4%
2. Scar rupture silent with tachycardia and scar tenderness	2. Scar rupture sudden with catastrophic clinical picture with more bleeding and shock
3. Scar dehiscence with less foetal mortality	3. Foetus and placenta usually thrown into peritoneal cavity hence foetal mortality very high
4. Usually occurs during active labour	4. Occurs even during pregnancy

weak and in such cases the decision for the trial of vaginal delivery should be well thought over.

5. *Presence of any other 'Risk factor':* A case of previous caesarean with any other risk factor or complication in current pregnancy such as malpresentation, APH, etc. is an indication for repeat caesarean section.

6. *In cases of doubtful pelvis or borderline CPD:* Trial labour is contraindicated. These cases should be for planned caesarean section.

7. *Tenderness on the scar:* If during the pregnancy or in labour, the area of the uterine scar is showing tenderness with unexplained tachycardia, indicating its weakness and proneness for rupture, then repeat caesarean should be performed immediately.

8. *Ultrasonography:* Tunneling of the scar is indicative of weakening of the scar. In such cases, caesarean section should be undertaken.

Under any circumstances, a previous caesarean case has to be delivered in a well-equipped institution having all the facilities for operative delivery, resuscitation of the mother and child and always under an expert supervision. The dictum therefore, changes as

Once a Caesarean, always a Hospital Delivery!

19

Obstetric Haemorrhage

OBSTETRIC HYSTERECTOMY

Sometimes hysterectomy becomes obligatory during pregnancy, after delivery or after pregnancy termination. It is performed as a maternal life saving procedure only.

Indications

1. *Uterine Rupture*

- Patient in serious state of shock
- Uterine tear irregularly ragged and difficult to repair.

2. *Caesarean Hysterectomy*

Hysterectomy may be required at the time of caesarean section. Its indications are:

- Atonic flabby uterus not responding to conservative line of treatment and giving rise to uncontrollable profuse haemorrhage
- Inadvertant lacerations of uterine vessels leading to furious haemorrhage
- Placenta accreta
- Severe intrauterine infection: It has become a rare indication since the introduction of wide spectrum antibiotics.
- Invasive carcinoma cervix
- Significant myomata preventing uterine contraction and causing haemorrhage.

3. *Following Vaginal Delivery*

- Atonic postpartum haemorrhage where conservative measures have failed

- Cases of morbidly adherent placenta where manual removal of placenta has failed on account of inability to obtain the plane of cleavage.

4. *Molar Pregnancy*

- Uncontrollable haemorrhage
- Serious trauma to the uterus during vaginal evacuation
- Prophylactic hysterectomy may be considered for age >40 years and/or parity >3 for fear of increased risk of choriocarcinoma.

5. *Abortions*

- Uncontrollable haemorrhage
- Severely damaged uterus
- Badly infected uterus–particularly in cases of criminal abortions.

Extent of Hysterectomy

Since these patients are in reproductive age group and young, usually total hysterectomy is performed leaving the ovaries behind. However, postpartum or caesarean hysterectomy is an emergency life saving procedure. Therefore, to save the time, subtotal hysterectomy may be performed, since it is technically easy and quick procedure with minimal chances of injury to urinary bladder, ureters or rectum.

When hysterectomy is indicated for carcinoma of cervix, radial hysterectomy is the procedure of choice.

Conservative Surgical Procedures for Management of PPH (Alternative to hysterectomy)

- Ligation of anterior division of internal iliac artery
- B-Lynch suture
- Stepwise devascularization

Ligation of Internal Iliac Artery

- Technically difficult procedure
- Successful in about 50% cases of postpartum hemorrhage

- Unilateral or bilateral ligation can be carried out as per the nature of bleeding.

Procedure

- Opening the peritoneum over the common iliac artery and dissecting down to its bifurcation into external and internal iliac artery.
- The areolar sheath covering the internal iliac artery is incised longitudinally.
- Right angle clamp is carefully passed just beneath the artery taking care not to injure the adjacent large veins. Non-absorbable suture is inserted into the open clamp, jaws are locked, suture is carried around the vessel and the vessel is securely ligated (Fig. 19.1).
- Pulsations of external iliac artery are checked.

Results

This results in 85% reduction in pulse pressure in arteries distal to the ligation. It converts arterial pressure system into that approaching venous circulation.

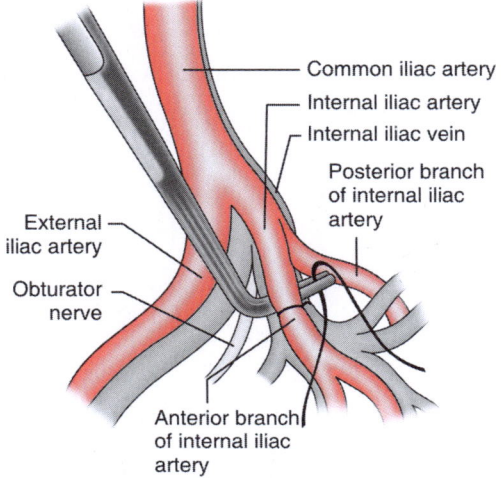

Fig. 19.1: Internal iliac artery ligation

Bilateral ligation does not appear to interfere with subsequent reproduction.

Precautions

Care to avoid injury to iliac vessels and ureters.

B-LYNCH SUTURE (Fig. 19.2)

- Laparotomy is done under GA and lower segment of anterior wall of the uterus is incised.
- Bimanual compression of uterus is tried first to assess the potential chance of success.
- Chromic catgut no. 2 suture is passed 3 cm below the lower edge on right side, is brought out 3 cm above the upper edge.
- The catgut is taken over the fundus of the uterus to the posterior aspect and posterior wall is pierced at the level of the incision to enter the uterine cavity. Now, the suture is brought out 3 cm above the upper edge of the incision.
- Again the catgut is taken over the anterior wall and the fundus to the posterior wall up to 3 cm below the level of incision and brought to anterior wall by piercing the uterus.
- The ends are tied strongly to squeeze the uterus.

VERTICAL UTERINE COMPRESSION SUTURES

This procedure has an advantage that these sutures can be placed without opening the uterus. These sutures can be taken

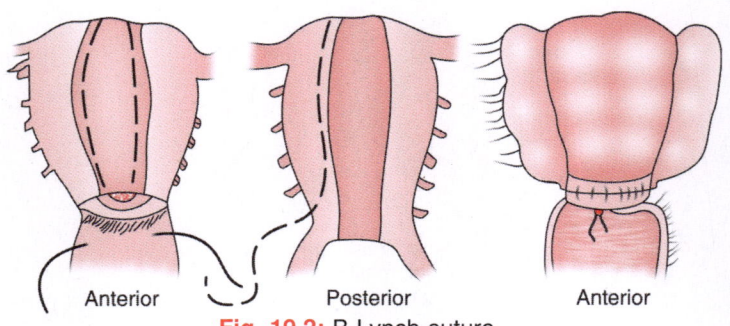

Anterior   Posterior   Anterior

Fig. 19.2: B-Lynch suture

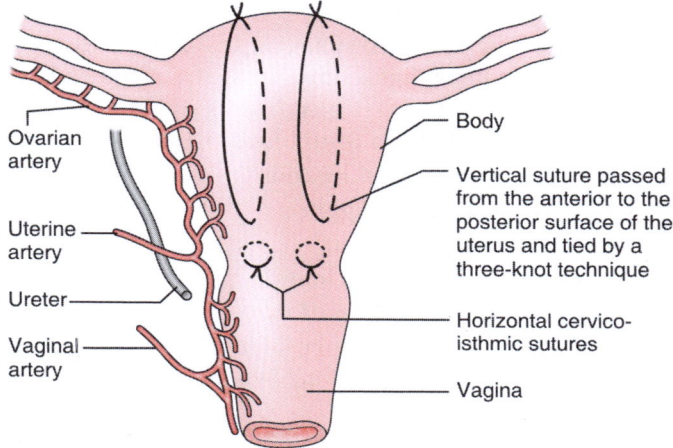

Fig. 19.3: Verticle uterine compression sutures

if no lower segment incision is present. Two vertical sutures as shown in the Fig. 19.3 are taken.

CHO MULTIPLE SQUARE COMPRESSION SUTURES

Multiple square sutures are taken at various places to cover the entire body of the uterus (Fig. 19.4). This is particularly very useful in placenta praevia.

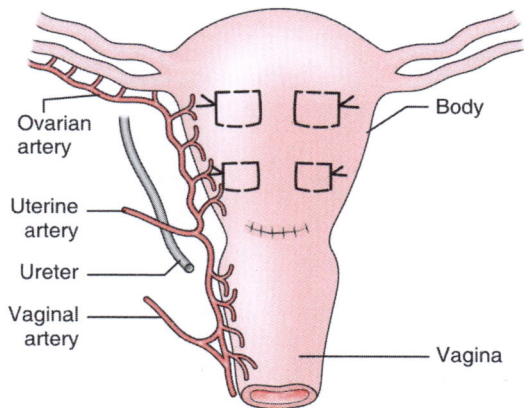

Fig.19.4: CHO multiple square compression sutures

STEPWISE UTERINE DEVASCULARIZATION

Stepwise uterine devascularization to control uncontrollable postpartum hemorrhage comprises of successive stepwise ligation of blood vessels. If bleeding is not controlled by one step the next step is taken until bleeding stops. The steps are:

1. Unilateral uterine vessel ligation
2. Bilateral uterine vessel ligation
3. Low uterine vessel ligation
4. Unilateral ovarian vessel ligation
5. Bilateral ovarian vessel ligation

This is claimed to be very effective procedure. More complicated procedure like internal iliac ligation may be avoided by this.

20

Destructive Operations

CRANIOTOMY

It is a surgical procedure wherein head is perforated to drain the brain matter to bring about the collapse of the foetal head. This reduces the size of the foetal head to effect the delivery that was obstructed by a large head.

Indications

1. *Hydrocephalus*: This is the only indication for this procedure in live foetus, however, tapping of the head by lumbar puncture needle mostly suffices here.
2. *Dead foetus with prolonged second stage* with deep transverse arrest/persistent occipitoposterior position leading to obstructed labour.
3. *Dead foetus with arrested aftercoming head* in breech delivery.

Anaesthesia

Pudendal block or short general anaesthesia.

Instruments

- Simpson's perforator (Fig. 20.1)
- Obstetric forceps/volsellum

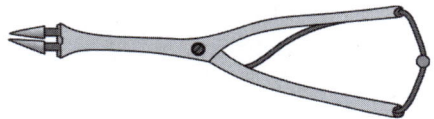

Fig. 20.1: Simpson's perforator

Prerequisites

- Baby must be dead.
- Head must be completely engaged; otherwise it has to be fixed from above so as to avoid its slipping and resulting into maternal injuries while perforating.
- Cervix must be fully dilated. But in cases of hydrocephalic head one should not wait till full dilatation of cervix, as there is danger of rupture of uterus.
- Bladder must be empty.
- Generous episiotomy should be given.

Procedure

1. *Steadying the head:* This is a very important step to avoid maternal injuries by the perforator due to slipping of the head. Head can be fixed by application of obstetric forceps, holding it with volsellum or in cases of large hydrocephalic foetus by holding it from above over the abdomen by an assistant.
2. *Incision:* An incision is taken on the scalp at the site selected for perforation.

Presentation	Site for perforation
Vertex	Near the bregma; but never in the fontanelle as it tends to close
Face/brow	Palate or orbit
Aftercoming head	Occipital bone close to posterolateral fontanelle.

3. *Perforation:* Simpson's perforator held in right hand with the blades closed is guided under a protecting left palm placed anterior to the selected site. A guiding hand anteriorly is essential to prevent accidental injury to the urinary bladder, in case the perforator slips. The blades are thrust into the skull bone to perforate. The blades are opened wide to widen the perforation. Again the blades are closed and locked; the perforator is then rotated through 90° and is opened again to widen the perforation further in vertical direction.
4. *Decompression of the head:* The brain matter is churned by moving the blades. Care is taken to reach right up to the

foramen magnum to destroy the basal nuclei; so that the baby will not take respiratory gasps after birth.

5. *Extraction:* The dead foetus is then extracted by giving traction on the forceps or the volsellum already applied.

Complications

- Bladder injury resulting in vesical fistulae
- Injury to the lower uterine segment
- Injury to the lower genital organs resulting into traumatic postpartum haemorrhage
- Failure to deliver the head

In modern obstetrics, there are very few instances like cases of borderline cephalopelvic disproportion where craniotomy is used for the delivery of the dead foetus. If the pelvis is grossly contracted, this procedure should not be attempted.

DECAPITATION

It is a procedure in which head of the foetus is severed from its trunk. The foetus is then extracted, first by its trunk and then the head.

Indication

Impacted shoulder with dead foetus, when its neck is easily accesible and cervix is fully dilated.

Instruments

- Blond-Heidler thimble and decapitating wire
- Decapitation knife or hook

Procedure

A. *Decapitation*

The Blond-Heidler thimble is mounted on the thumb and decapitation wire is attached to it. The whole hand is inserted into the vagina. The thumb is then passed in front of the neck and the fingers behind to pull the thimble with the attached wire round the foetal neck.

The ends of wire are then mounted on the handles and foetal neck is severed by to and fro movement of the wire. This method is safer than the use of decapitation knife or hook.

Alternatively

By exerting pressure on the prolapsed arm, the neck is brought within easy access. The decapitation hook protected by palm of left hand is passed over the foetal neck. The knife is carried through the foetal neck by its backward and forward movement.

B. *Delivery*

After the head is completely severed, the trunk is delivered by traction on the arm. The severed head is then delivered manually by a finger hooked in the mouth and pulling on the jaw or with the forceps.

Risk

Injury to the maternal soft parts, resulting in traumatic postpartum haemorrhage or fistulae, specially due to the bony spicules at the ragged severed neck or due to the instrument.

EVISCERATION

It is a procedure to remove abdominal and thoracic contents of the dead foetus for reducing its bulk, facilitating its easy extraction.

Indication

Impacted shoulder presentation with dead foetus, where foetal abdomen is easily accessible.

Instrument

Embryotomy scissors, which are much stouter than normal surgical scissors.

Procedure

1. Foetal trunk is steadied by pulling on the prolapsed arm.

2. A large opening is made with the help of embryotomy scissors in the foetal abdomen or thorax.
3. Viscera are broken up and removed manually. If the opening is made in thorax, then abdominal viscera are reached through the diaphragm.
4. After removal of the viscera, the foetus collapses and can be delivered easily by giving traction on the prolapsed arm.

In modern obstetrics, caesarean section is performed in cases of impacted shoulder presentation with dead foetus on account of its greater safety.

CLEIDOTOMY

This is a procedure of division of the clavicles by means of the embryotomy scissors to reduce the bulk of shoulder girdle.

Indication

Shoulder dystocia with dead foetus. (Often encountered in macrosomic infants of diabetic mothers.)

Instrument

Embryotomy scissors

Procedure

Both the clavicles are divided by embryotomy scissors introduced under the protection of left hand.

Risk

Injury to maternal soft parts either by severed foetal bony spicules or by the instrument.

21

Manual Removal of Placenta

Manual removal of placenta is performed when the placenta fails to deliver naturally in the third stage of labour.

Indications

1. If separation and expulsion of placenta has not resulted within 30 minutes of the birth of the foetus.
2. If there is dangerous amount of bleeding in third stage of labour and if routine measures of delivering the placenta have failed.

Causes of Retension

- Trapped placenta
- Simple adhesion
- *Morbid adhesion:* Accreta, increta, percreta

Anaesthesia

In this procedure, the whole hand is to be introduced inside the uterus. The uterus therefore has to be completely relaxed. Hence, this procedure has to be performed under deep general anaesthesia–*ether or halothane.*

Procedure

1. Before actual procedure is started
   - IV drip is kept running.
   - Cross-matched blood is kept ready.
   - Urinary bladder is emptied.
2. Patient is given lithotomy position, painted and draped.

3. The cord is held taught with left hand and right hand is introduced into the uterus. After entering the uterine cavity, the cord is followed up to the edge of the placenta.

4. The fundus of the uterus is steadied with the left hand on the abdomen while the assistant is asked to hold the cord taught.

5. Having reached the lower margin of the placenta, membranes are pushed under the margin of the placenta. The placenta is separated with a sweeping movement of the hand. External hand moves the fundus to facilitate these manipulations.

6. When the placenta is separated completely, it is manoeuvred on the palm of right hand. Then by pulling on the cord, the placenta is slided alongside the wrist, leaving the right hand inside the uterine cavity to feel for the remnants of the placental tissue and for any rent in the uterus, thus avoiding the need for reintroduction of the hand.

7. After completing the procedure:
   - Administration of anaesthetic agent is discontinued.
   - Intravenous injection of oxytocics is given.
   - Adequate blood transfusion to replace the blood loss.
   - Broad spectrum antibiotics to prevent infection.

Failure to get the plane of cleavage and thus to separate the placenta indicates morbid adhesion of placenta. In such cases:

1. Try to remove as much placenta as possible.

2. If few bits are left inside the uterus which do not cause significant bleeding:
   - Antibiotics
   - Methotrexate

3. If significant bleeding, then hysterectomy has to be performed.

Complications of MRP

During Procedure

- Shock
- Cardiac arrest

- Severe haemorrhage
- Perforation of the uterine wall by fingers.

Immediate Postoperative

- Shock
- Haemorrhage
- Sepsis
- Pelvic thrombophlebitis.

Delayed

- Weakening of the uterine wall leading to rupture in subsequent pregnancy.
- Third stage complications like PPH and retention of placenta in subsequent pregnancies.

MTP and Family Planning

22. MTP Act

23. MTP Procedures

24. Natural Methods of Contraception

25. Barrier Contraception

26. Hormonal Contraception

27. Intrauterine Contraceptive Devices

28. Female Sterilization

29. Male Sterilization

MTP Act

After considering the report of Shantilal Shah Commission, MTP act 1971 was implemented in India from 1st April, 1972. According to the Act, Medical Termination of pregnancy is legalised in our country to bring down the Maternal and Child mortality and morbidity. The MTP Rules were first modified in 1975. The Act has been amended in 2002. The MTP Rules are published in the official gazette on 13 June 2003.

Who can get Aborted?

Legal limit for MTP is 20 weeks of pregnancy.

Indications

1. If the current pregnancy is likely to
   - Endanger woman's life
   - Cause grave injury to her physical or mental health
2. If the child born is likely to suffer from any mental or physical disability so as to render it seriously handicapped.
3. If the pregnancy is caused by rape.
4. If the pregnancy has resulted due to contraceptive failure.
5. If actual or reasonably foreseen social or economic environments are likely to cause risk to her physical or mental health.

Who can Perform MTP?

Registered medical practitioner (RMP) fulfilling any of the following conditions:
- Who is having postgraduate qualification (degree or diploma) in obstetrics and gynaecology

- Who has minimum of six months experience as resident medical officer, house surgeon or postgraduate student in the department of obstetrics and gynaecology?
- Who has assisted a registered medical practitioner in the performance of 25 cases of MTP of which at least five have been performed independently, in a hospital established or maintained, or a training institute approved for this purpose by the Government? This training would enable the practitioner to perform first trimester terminations only.
- Those Registered Medical Practitioners who have registered themselves before 1971 and have experience of at least three years medical practice in the field of obstetrics and gynaecology.
- Those who have registered themselves as medical practitioner after 1971 and who bear the experience of medical practice in the field of obstetrics and gynaecology for minimum one year.

Where can MTP be Performed?

MTP should be performed in an authorized MTP centre. Upon receipt of an application in form A, the chief medical officer of the district will inspect the place to see whether it is safe and hygienic for performing MTP. He will then recommend the approval of such place to the district committee. The committee will then give the approval in form B. The certificate of approval shall be conspicuously displayed at the place to be easily visible to persons visiting the place.

The Prerequisites for MTP Centre

For up to 12 weeks:
- Gynecology examination/labour table
- Equipment for resuscitation
- Facilities for sterilization of instruments
- Emergency drugs and parenteral fluids
- Back up facilities for treatment of shock and facilities for transportation

For up to 20 weeks:
- Well equipped operation theatre to perform abdominal and gynecological surgery
- Anesthetic equipment, resuscitation and sterilization equipment
- Drugs and parenteral fluids in sufficient supply for emergency use.

For medical abortion using mifepristone

Prescription of mifepristone/misoprostol can be given by the RMP at his clinic provided he/she has access to an approved place for MTP. The RMP should display a certificate to this effect from the owner of the approved place.

Admission Register

Record of MTP patient must be maintained in a separate and special register. Patient's name appears only in this register. On the case papers and other hospital and operation theatre registers, only patient's MTP number appears. This MTP register is to be kept in safe custody of the owner of the hospital for minimum five years from the date of last entry in the register.

Consent for MTP

The consent has to be obtained on a separately prescribed consent form (form C). If the patient is above the age of 18 years then her own consent is obtained; but if she is minor or mentally ill the consent of her legal guardian has to be sought for.

Opinion for Performing MTP

For first trimester MTP, opinion of only one doctor authorized to perform MTP is sufficient, but for second trimester MTP, two such doctors have to certify the necessity of MTP. These opinions are to be signed on a specially prescribed form (Form I).

The consent form and the intimation form are placed in an envelop which has to be sealed and marked 'Secret'. The owner or head of the hospital has to preserve these envelopes containing forms in safe custody.

Monthly Report

The monthly report of MTPs done in the hospital has to be submitted in form II to the chief medical officer of the state.

Secrecy

The institution and doctor; both are legally bound to observe the confidentiality for the MTP performed; failing which, they are liable for prosecution.

Methods of MTP are classified into two groups according to period of pregnancy. The methods of first trimester MTP are easy, less time consuming and carry lesser risk of complications.

A. Methods for First Trimester MTP

1. Medical method
   - Mifepristone–Misoprostol sequential administration
2. Surgical methods
   - Menstrual regulation
   - Suction evacuation
     Manual vacuum aspiration (MVA)
     Electric vacuum aspiration (EVA)
   - Dilatation and evacuation

B. Methods for Second Trimester MTP

1. Medicosurgical methods
   - Extra-amniotic methods
     - Ethacridine lactate
     - Prostaglandins
     - Simple rubber catheter
2. Medical method
   - Prostaglandins
3. Surgical methods
   - Abdominal hysterotomy

MEDICAL ABORTION

Mifepristone and Misopristol are administered sequentially in this method.

189

Mifepristone

- Synthetic 19–norsteroid with high affinity for progesterone receptors, but very little progestational activity
- Mode of action:
  - It blocks the effect of progesterone on the target tissue, i.e. endometrium; resulting in sloughing of decidual tissue; thus causing early abortion.
  - Decidual PG synthesis is increased and PG catabolism is decreased leading to decidual necrosis with bleeding and detachment of embryo.
  - This leads to fall in trophoblastic β-HCG production resulting in reduced progesterone production from corpus luteum.
  - Causes marked increase in myometrial sensitivity to exogenously administered prostaglandins.
  - Softens the uterine cervix

Misoprostol

- PGE_1 analogue available as 200 µg tablets for oral use. These tablets can be administered vaginally with more potent oxytocic effect.
- Mode of action: Due to its potent oxytocic action
  - Stimulates uterine contractions
  - Causes cervical softening

Use for Medical Abortion

Mifepristone used alone has low efficacy. Severe uterine haemorrhage is known. Its combination with prostaglandins is shown to increase the efficacy and safety. Hence, sequential administration of Mifepristone/Misoprostol has been recommended. This medical method is approved in India for medical termination of early pregnancy up to 9 weeks (63 days).

Method of Administration

- Day 1–Mifepristone 200 mg orally
- Day 3–Misoprostol 400 µg orally up to 7 weeks of pregnancy
  Misoprostol 800 µg vaginally up to 9 weeks of pregnancy

- Day 14–Post-treatment evaluation
- Efficacy 90–95%

Contraindications

- Confirmed or suspected ectopic pregnancy or undiagnosed adnexal mass.
- Chronic adrenal failure
- Concurrent long-term corticosteroid therapy
- History of allergy to mifepristone, misoprostol or other prostaglandin
- Hemorrhagic disorders or concurrent anticoagulant therapy
- Inherited porphyrias

Information to Patients

- The necessity of completing the treatment schedule, including a follow-up visit
- Vaginal bleeding and uterine cramping may occur for 7–14 days
- Efficacy up to 95%
- If the treatment fails, there is a risk of fetal malformation
- Medical abortion treatment failures are managed by surgical termination.

METHODS FOR FIRST TRIMESTER MTP

MENSTRUAL REGULATION

This method was used for terminating very early pregnancy; within a fortnight after missing the period. It does not require dilatation of the cervix and hence any anaesthesia.

Instruments

- *Karman cannula:* These cannulae are available in different sizes, from 4 mm diameter. Their length is 22 cm. They have two eyes near the tip (Fig. 23.1).

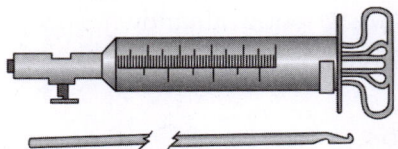

Fig. 23.1: Menstrual regulation syringe and Karman cannula

Menstrual regulation syringe comprises:
1. Plastic syringe of 50 ml capacity
2. Piston with rubber stopper and two flanges
3. Plastic valve to create negative pressure
4. Rubber valve liner

Sterilization of the MR Kit

- Karman cannulae are available as disposable gamma rays presterilized packs.
- MR syringe with all its parts is to be sterilized by chemical method (2% glutaraldehyde) or in formalin chamber for minimum 20 minutes.

Steps of Operation

1. Patient is given lithotomy position after voiding urine.
2. Cervix is visualized with Sim's speculum and anterior vaginal wall retractor and anterior lip is caught by volsellum.
3. Karman cannula of appropriate size is introduced through the cervical canal into the uterine cavity.
4. The valve at the nozzle of the MR syringe is closed and the piston is pulled out till the flanges by the side of the piston rest on the collar of the syringe.
5. The Karman cannula in situ is attached to the rubber valve liner and the valve is opened.
6. Negative pressure inside the MR syringe aspirates the products of conception. They are indentified from the blood clots by their whitish appearance.
7. Sensation of grating at the tip of the Karman cannula and the bloody foam in it, indicate that the aspiration is complete.

8. Aspirated material can be sent for histopathological study for confirmation of pregnancy

Advantages
1. No anaesthesia and no hospitalization
2. No assistance is required
3. Economical
4. Minimal bleeding
5. Minimal risk of complications
6. No need for confirmation of pregnancy.

Disadvantages
1. Unsuitable for pregnancy beyond 6 weeks
2. The chances of failure of procedure are more in comparison to other methods.

Complications

1. Uterine perforation
2. Infection
3. Post-abortal haemorrage in cases of incomplete aspiration
4. Failure to aspirate the gestational sac is known. In such cases the pregnancy may continue.
5. Rarely, tip of Karman cannula may break inside if the cannula is used repeatedly.

Other use of MR Syringe

For endometrial biopsy.

MANUAL VACUUM ASPIRATION (MVA)

Currently double valve kits (Table 23.1) are available for MVA which consist of:

- 60 ml syringe with double locking valve, plunger handle and collar stop, made of high density polypropylene (Fig. 23.2).
- Sterile flexible cannulae–3 to 12 mm sizes, made of high density polypropylene and a set of adaptors to fit each cannula to the syringe. Cannulae and adaptors are color coded to fit into the double valve adapter (Fig. 23.3).

Table 23.1: Single valve and double valve aspirators

Single valve aspirator	Double valve aspirator
One valve	Two valves
Up to 6 mm cannulae used	Up to 12 mm cannulae used
MTP up to 6 weeks	MTP up to 12 weeks
50 ml capacity syringe	60 ml capacity syringe
Vaccum maintained till 50% full	Till 80% full

The double valve syringe and the cannulae can be used for vacuum aspiration of uterine cavity up to 10–12 weeks of uterine size. The procedure is carried out under local paracervical anesthesia.

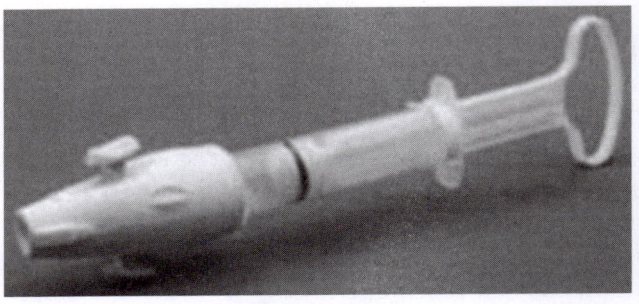

Fig. 23.2: MVA syringe

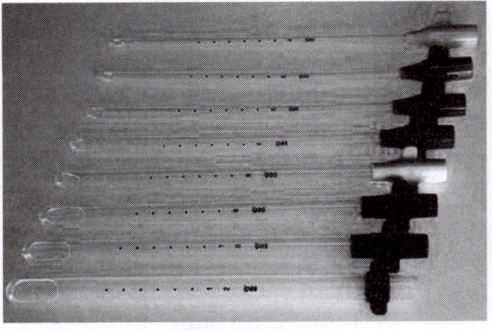

Fig. 23.3: MVA cannulae

Steps

- Create vacuum in the syringe.
- Perform bimanual examination and note the uterine size
- Give paracervical anesthesia
- Dilate the cervix with cannulae, dilators or Misoprostol pretreatment
- Insert the selected cannula through the cervix
- Attach the syringe and release the valves
- Rotate the cannula in the uterine cavity to aspirate the contents
- Look for signs of completeness
- Inspect the evacuated material

Advantage

Simple, cheap, portable device, safe procedure suited for rural set up, no electricity required, OPD procedure. Can be used for endometrial aspiration also.

Table 23.2: MVA vs medical abortion	
Vacuum aspiration	*Medical abortion*
Surgical technique using elctrical/manual suction instruments	Non surgical technique using drugs
Cannula attached to handheld vacuum syringe or electric pump	Mifepristone–antiprogestin, Misoprostol–PG used sequentially
Can be done up to 12 weeks of pregnancy	Can be done up to 9 weeks of pregnancy in India
More than 98% effective	90–95% effective
15–20 minutes to complete the procedure	May take 9–16 days for complete abortion to occur
POC examined and confirmed immediately	POC may be expelled at home
Single visit	At least 3 visits
Repeat VA for failures	VA if failed procedure
Local anesthesia	No anesthesia
Risk of cervical and uterine injury	No risk of cervical and uterine injury
Post procedure pain and bleeding less	Prolonged post procedure pain and bleeding

ELECTRICAL VACUUM ASPIRATION (SUCTION EVACUATION)

This method is used for terminating first trimester pregnancy. This method requires the dilatation of the cervix and hence some anaesthesia.

Instruments

- Instruments for cervical dilatation
- *A set of suction cannulae:* These cannulae are of different sizes, ranging from diameters 4 mm to 12 mm (Fig. 23.4).
  The cannulae are provided with uterine curve with two eyes at the tip to suck in the products of conception. At the proximal end of cannula there is a small aperture valve which can be operated by thumb to maintain or release vacuum in the system. Usually these are metal cannulae, however plastic cannulae are also available.
- *Suction machine:* Electric or foot operated with capacity to produce suction up to 0.8 kg/cm^2. The force of suction required for termination of pregnancy is 625 mm of Hg.
- *Tube to connect the cannula to the suction bottle:* This is tough enough not to collapse by the atmospheric pressure after production of negative pressure.

Anaesthesia

Pericervical, paracervical or general.

Steps of Operation

1. Patient is given lithotomy position.
2. Per vaginal examination is carried out to determine the size and position of the uterus.
3. The cervix is visualized and its anterior lip is caught with volsellum and anaesthesia is given.
4. Cervix is dilated gradually by cervical dilators. The extent of dilatation should be 1 mm more than the size of cannula.

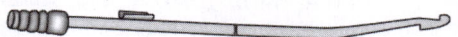

Fig. 23.4: Suction cannula

5. Suction cannula of desired size is inserted into the uterus up to the fundus. Usually the number of cannula to be used corresponds to the weeks of gestation. The curvature of the cannula is directed according to the position of the uterus.

6. The negative pressure in the suction is created up to 0.8 kg/cm^2 or 625 mm of Hg with its valve closed.

7. Cannula with its tip inside the uterine cavity is attached to the suction bottle with the help of a tube.

8. Air inlet valve on the shoulder of the cannula is closed by thumb, suction valve is opened and the cannula is slowly rotated around itself. Products of conception are aspirated in an airtight suction bottle.

9. Grating sensation, gripping of the cannula by contracting uterus confirm the completion of the abortion. Then the cannula is withdrawn.

Advantages

1. Short procedure; hence less bleeding
2. Safe method up to 12 weeks of gestation
3. Risk of complications is low.

Disadvantages

1. Requires skilled surgeon.
2. An assistant is required to handle the suction apparatus.
3. Chances of incomplete evacuation.
4. Consequences of perforations are grave.
5. Anaesthesia is required.
6. If done under general anaesthesia, hospitalization for at least four hours is required.

Table 23.3: Comparison of MVA and EVA	
MVA	*EVA*
Portable, economical, hand held	Expensive, heavy, equipment, requires electricity
Suited for rural setting	Suited for urban setting
Quick creation of vacuum, vacuum loaded syringe	Takes couple of minutes
In case of uterine perforation vacuum drops to <10 mm of Hg hence viscera not aspirated	In case of perforation vaccum continues to aspirate, visceral tissues likely to get aspirated

DILATATION AND EVACUATION

Dilatation and evacuation is by far the oldest method used for termination of pregnancy. Currently not used on account of the complications.

There are two methods of dilatation of the cervix; slow dilatation and rapid dilatation.

Rapid dilatation is achieved by means of metal dilators like Hegar's dilators. Being a painful procedure anaesthesia is necessary.

Currently, prostaglandin preparations (Misoprostol or PGF_2-α) are used for cervical softening and dilatation before MTP.

Slow dilatation is achieved by hygroscopic tents like laminaria tents or isapgol tents. These tents absorb moisture from the tissues due to their hygroscopic action and swell to open the cervix. This is painless procedure not requiring anaesthesia. It requires about 4 hours for the desired action. This method is not used currently.

Anaesthesia

General, pericervical or paracervical.

Instruments

- Instruments for D & C
- Ovum forceps

Steps of Operation

Depending upon the size of the ovum forceps, the cervix is gradually dilated-usually up to no. 14. Ovum forceps is introduced into the uterine cavity slowly and carefully. Products of conception are removed by ovum forceps. Uterine cavity is curetted by blunt curette. The empty uterus gives grating sensation through the curette.

Advantage

Chances of abortion remaining incomplete are less.

Disadvantages

In comparison to suction evacuation:

- Prolonged procedure; hence more bleeding.
- High incidence of perforation with injury to viscera.

COMPLICATIONS OF SURGICAL PROCEDURES OF FIRST TRIMESTER MTP

The surgical methods of first trimester MTP involve forceful dilatation of the cervix and evacuation of the uterine cavity. The complications of all these methods are therefore, the same, only the gravity, extent and incidence change according to the method.

Immediate	*Delayed*
Uterine perforation	Cervical incompetence
Cervical lacerations	Tubal block
Haemorrhage	Aschermann's syndrome
Infection	

UTERINE PERFORATION

Uterine perforation can take place at any stage of the procedure. Sound, dilators, ovum forceps, curette, Karman cannula or suction cannula–any of these instruments can cause perforation during their use. Pregnant uterus being softer and larger than the nonpregnant uterus, chances of perforation in these procedures are more in comparison to dilatation and curettage performed in nonpregnant uteri.

How to Suspect and Diagnose Uterine Perforation?

a. The instrument in use unexpectedly escapes inside the uterine cavity–more than what it was going previously.

b. Resistance of the uterine musculature is not felt at the tip of the instrument.

c. After suspecting the perforation, when uterine sound is passed in the uterine cavity, it goes in more than the expected length of the uterus.

d. Suddenly, excessive bleeding may start from the uterine cavity.

e. Ovum forceps may pull out omentum, a loop of intestine or rarely, fallopian tube.

Management of Uterine Perforation

The first and most important principle in managing the uterine perforation is to stop the procedure immediately. Further management depends upon whether any visceral organ has been brought out through the perforation or not and whether the abortion is complete or incomplete (Flow chart 23.1).

No Visceral Injury

A. *Evacualtion Complete*

1. Send the blood for grouping and cross-matching.
2. Start IV dextrose 5%.
3. Start suitable broad spectrum antibiotics.
4. Admit the patient in the wards and keep a close watch on pallor, pulse rate, blood pressure, type and rate of respiration, abdominal girth, intestinal peristalsis and vaginal bleeding.
5. If any of the above parameters indicate deterioration, laparotomy is indicated for suturing the uterine rent.

   Signs of internal bleeding:
   - Persistent or increasing tachycardia (pulse >100/min) is suggestive of excessive haemorrhage, which can be vaginal bleeding or bleeding in the peritoneal cavity.
   - Blood pressure <100 mm of Hg systolic
   - Increasing pallor
   - Abdominal distension with signs of free fluid.
6. If the perforation gets sealed by itself, there is no significant change in vital parameters. If the patient remains stable after 24 hours, she can be discharged from the hospital.

B. *Incomplete Evacuation*

If abortion is incomplete, then it is to be completed, but blind per vaginal intervention may worsen the damage. In such cases, completion of abortion vaginally under laparoscopic control is possible. But where laparoscopic facility is not available, laparotomy is indicated for evacuation of the uterus.

Flow Chart 23.1: Management of uterine perforation

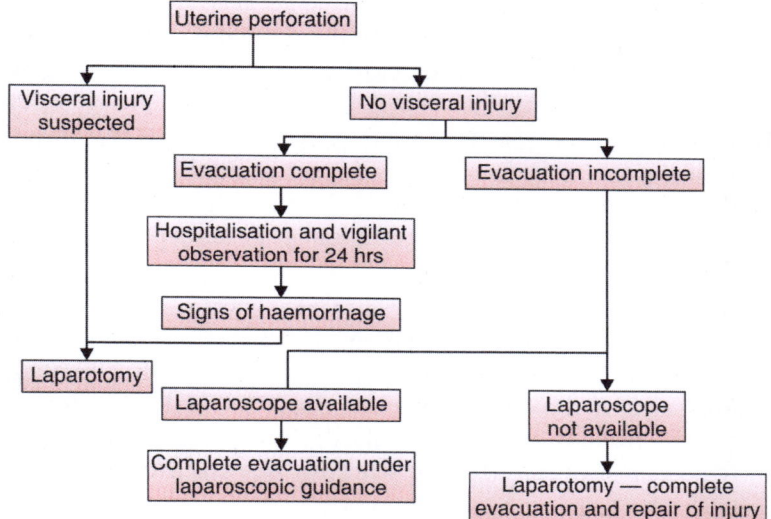

Visceral Injury

- If any of the visceral organs is pulled out, then there is no place for conservative line of treatment. An immediate laparotomy should be performed in such cases.
- If the perforation has occurred by suction cannula with suction on, intestines or omentum is likely to be sucked in and damaged; hence laparotomy is usually indicated.
- Increasing abdominal girth with absent peristalsis are indicative of haemorrhage, peritonitis or overlooked intestinal injury. Hence, laparotomy should be performed.

CERVICAL LACERATIONS

Usually difficult forceful dilatation of cervix against considerable resistance causes cervical lacerations. If the lacerations are minimal, they might be left alone. But if the cervical injury is large with alarming bleeding then surgical repair is indicated. Sometimes excessive bleeding through minor tear can be tackled by cauterization or tight packing of the vagina.

HAEMORRHAGE

Aetiology

a. If the procedure is unduly prolonged, then the incompletely evacuated uterus cannot contract properly resulting in excessive bleeding.

b. *Incomplete evacuation:* Completion of the abortion is required. When examined, these cases reveal dilated cervical canal through which the products of conception may be felt. Occasionally, patient may complain of passing products and the bleeding continues.

c. *Uterine perforation:* Vide supra

d. *Uterine atony :* The uterus remains flabby and starts bleeding heavily. IV, oxytocin drip or IM. Prostodin is given. Bimanual massage of the uterus is also done to facilitate uterine contraction. If all these methods fail, then occasionally, hysterectomy may be required for saving the life of the patient.

e. *Infection:* Vide infra.

The management of these cases consists of treatment of the cause of the haemorrhage and replacement of the blood loss.

INFECTION

Aetiology

a. Failure to observe proper aseptic precautions

b. Incomplete evacuation can lead to ascending infections.

c. Preexisting subclinical infection may become overt after surgical procedure.

Diagnosis

- Foul smelling discharge per vaginum.
- Fever
- Pain in the hypogastric region
- Tenderness in lower abdomen and in pelvis.
- Excessive vaginal bleeding.

Treatment

Appropriate use of antibiotics is the main line of treatment. However, if the infection is due to incomplete abortion, evacuation of uterus under antibiotics cover is essential.

CERVICAL INCOMPETENCE

Due to forceful rapid dilatation of the cervix, few fibers of the circular muscles are torn resulting in cervical incompetence. This can be avoided by use of prostaglandins or by cervical tents. Menstrual regulation procedure performed in earlier weeks is free from this complication as it does not require cervical dilatation.

TUBAL BLOCK

Usually this is the sequelae of post MTP pelvic infection.

INTRAUTERINE SYNAECHIAE

Due to vigourous curettage, basal endometrium is removed leaving raw area open in the uterine cavity. This leads to the formation of adhesions or synaechiae. This is known as Aschermann's syndrome.

Considering these delayed complications, as far as possible, primigravid patients are discouraged from surgical MTP.

METHODS FOR SECOND TRIMESTER MTP

EXTRA-AMNIOTIC METHODS

The commonly used drug for second trimester MTP is Ethacridine lactate. Alternatively 15 methyl PGF$_2$-α can also be used by this route.

EXTRA-AMNIOTIC INSTILLATION OF ETHACRIDINE LACTATE

Indications

1. MTP in second trimester.
2. Termination of pregnancy in cases of:
   - Missed abortion when the pregnancy is more than 12 weeks.

- Intrauterine foetal death and diagnosed foetal anomalies like anencephaly, hydrocephaly, etc.

Mode of Action

- Oxytocic action due to the release of prostaglandins
- Mechanical stimulation of the uterus by the drug and the catheter
- Oxytocic effect of the drug

Instruments

- Instruments for visualization of cervix
- Foley's catheter no. 16 or 18
- Syringe (20 CC or 50 CC) with needle
- Ethacridine lactate 0.1% (150 ml)

Procedure

1. Cervix is visualized and caught by volsellum.
2. Sterilized Foley's catheter is introduced through the cervical canal (Magill's forceps may be used for this).
3. Bulb of the catheter is inflated by 10 ml of saline or distilled water.
4. Ethacridine lactate is instilled inside the uterine cavity in extra-amniotic space.
5. The distal end of the catheter is closed by an artery forceps or a string of thread.
6. The catheter is left inside and the patient is advised bed rest in order to avoid the leakage of the drug.
7. After 4 to 6 hours the catheter is removed after deflating the bulb.
8. If the patient fails to abort even after 72 hours; reinstillation of the drug is done.

Dose of the Ethacridine Lactate

- 150 ml (0.1%)
- 10 ml (0.1%) per week of pregnancy, not exceeding 150 ml.

Success Rate

80% to 85% cases abort within 72 hours of first instillation. Almost 100% cases abort after second instillation.

Induction–Abortion Interval

Usually 24 to 48 hours, with a mean interval of 36 hours. Augmentation by oxytocin or prostaglandins can reduce the interval.

Advantages
1. Wide margin of safety
2. No danger to the life even if the drug enters the maternal circulation
3. Potent and widespread bactericidal activity of the drug
4. Simple technique
5. No special contraindications
6. No scar on the uterus nor on the abdomen

Disadvantages
1. Failure in 10% to 15% patients at first instillation which prolongs the induction abortion interval.
2. Incomplete abortion leaving the placenta inside the uterus requires surgical evacuation.

Bleeding through the cervix: Low lying placenta may be disturbed by the catheter.

MEDICAL METHODS

15 METHYL PGF_2-α

This drug has been effectively used for second trimester MTPs intramuscular injection: 250 µg 3 hourly maximum 30 hrs.

Advantages
- Nonsurgical method
- Usable at all gestational ages
- Easy administration even by paramedical staff

Disadvantage
Gastrointestinal side effects

This drug has been used by intra-amniotic and extra-amniotic routes also. However, intramuscular administration is simpler.

Actions

- Stimulation of uterine contractions
- Softening and dilatation of cervix
- Leuteolytic effect

Advantages

- High success rate specially with intramuscular and intra-amniotic routes of administration
- Induction abortion interval is shorter in comparison to other methods for second trimester abortions–18 to 20 hours with cut-off time of 30 hours
- Effective at all stages of pregnancy

Disadvantages

- Costly medicine
- Troublesome side effects

Side Effects

- Gastrointestinal upsets–diarrhoea, vomiting
- Pyrexia and shivering

Complications

- High incidence of incomplete abortion requiring surgical evacuation
- Cervical injury sometimes leading to cervicovaginal fistulae.

Contraindications

- *Systemic diseases:* Bronchial asthma, hypertension, cardiac diseases, severe renal or liver diseases
- Scarred uterus
- Diarrhoea and dysentery

Mifepristone: Misoprostol sequential administration and Misoprostol alone are also being used for nonsurgical second trimester MTPs. However, in India, these drugs are not yet approved for second trimester MTP.

ABDOMINAL HYSTEROTOMY

It is a major abdominal surgical procedure. The overall mortality and morbidity associated with hysterotomy is quite high in comparison with less invasive and safer methods available today. Moreover, the scar on the uterus increases the risk of childbirth in subsequent pregnancies. Hence, it is used less frequently in modern obstetrics. This method is used only when other methods fail or are contraindicated, and abortion is obligatory.

Indications
- Placenta previa covering internal os of the cervix
- Pregnancy with carcinoma of cervix where hysterotomy has to be performed by classical incision
- Ovarian cyst requiring removal along with MTP.

Anaesthesia
Spinal, epidural or general.

Steps of Operation
1. Small transverse incision is taken on the lower uterine segment
2. The uterine cavity is emptied
3. Uterine wall is sutured
4. Abdominal wall is closed in layers.

24 | Natural Methods of Contraception

Contraceptive methods which do not require any medication or appliances are natural family planning methods.

FERTILITY AWARENESS BASED METHODS

Physiological Principles

- Menstrual cycle begins on the first day of the period and ends when the next period begins. Usual duration of cycle is 28 days.
- Ovulation takes place 13–14 days prior to next menstrual period in a regularly menstruating woman.
- Few days prior to ovulation there is excessive secretion of cervical mucous which is thinner, profuse and having a spinnbarkeit more than 10 cm. This is due to preovulatory high levels of oestrogen. Such mucous is having very good sperm penetration quality.
- After the ovulation, the mucous becomes scanty, thick and the spinnbarkeit less than 4 cm. Such mucous is having poor sperm penetration.
- Soon after ovulation, basal body temperature rises about 0.6° to 0.8° F and remains elevated until few days prior to the onset of next menstruation.

Based on these physiological principles, the woman identifies her own fertile period during which she avoids sexual contact or uses barrier methods.

Advantages
- Natural; therefore no side effects or complications
- Inexpensive

- Can be used throughout the reproductive period
- No drug, no device
- Acceptable to some religious groups which discourage use of other methods
- Enables all pregnancies to be planned
- These methods are also useful for the couples intending to have conception.

Disadvantages
- High motivation is needed
- Training is necessary
- Untoward effects of late fertilization
    - Aging gametes–congenital malformations
    - Ectopic pregnancy
    - Placenta praevia
- Unsuitable method for women with irregular periods
- Unsuitable for uneducated people
- Failure rate 10–30% which can be reduced by barrier methods during unsafe period.

RHYTHM METHOD (CALENDAR METHOD)

A week on both the sides of the day of ovulation is considered as unsafe period.

Considering the length of previous 6 menstrual cycles, shortest and longest cycles are identified.
- (Shortest cycle – 18) = first day of fertile period
- (Longest cycle – 11) = last day of fertile period

Disadvantages
- High failure rate
- Eventually reduces the safe period for intercourse
- Unsuitable for women with irregular cycles.

BASAL BODY TEMPERATURE (BBT) METHOD

Time of ovulation is detected by biphasic temperature chart and unprotected sex is avoided in periovulatory period.

Method

- Record BBT every morning before getting out of bed
- Couple should avoid unprotected sex up to 3 days after the temperature rise.

Limitation

- This method can identify the end but not the start of fertile period.
- Temperature may rise due to other factors.
- Some cycles may remain monophasic and still be ovulatory.

CERVICAL SECRETIONS TO IDENTIFY FERTILE PERIOD (BILLING'S METHOD)
Method

- Everyday woman checks for any cervical secretions at the vulva on her finger or tissue paper.
- As soon as she notices any secretions, unprotected sex is avoided.
- *Peak day:* Secretions are profuse, most slippery, stretchy and wet.
- Fourth day after the peak day the couple can have unprotected sex.

Disadvantages
- Vaginal fluid or semen could be confused with secretions.
- Spermicides, vaginal infections and some drugs also affect the pattern of secretions.

Instructions for BOM

Avoid intercourse from the appearance of the mucous till the peak day, i.e. last day of slippery, sticky, lubricate mucous; +3 days thereafter.

SYMPTOTHERMAL METHOD

This is combination of BBT and cervical mucous methods.

Woman avoids unprotected sex from the day, she senses cervical secretions till 4th day after peak cervical secretions and third day after rise of BBT.

LACTATIONAL AMENORRHOEA METHOD

Exclusive breastfeeding 8–10 times day (day and night) can provide contraception so long as the woman is amenorrhoic.

In response to nipple stimulation during lactation, prolactin secretion increases 2–20 folds in plasma within 5–15 minutes having half life in plasma for 10–30 minutes.

Mode of Action

- High prolactin levels inhibits LH (no effect on FSH)
- Partially inhibits ovarian response to both these gonadotropins.
- Inhibitory effect depends upon the frequency of nursing and duration of lactation.

Antifertility Effects of Prolactin

- Anovulation or erratic ovulation
- Short luteal phase
- Corpus luteal insufficiency–interference with implantation

The efficacy is more only till the woman gets her first menstruation following delivery, or the baby is exclusively breastfed day and night (started on complementary feeding) or up to 4 months.

Failure in first six months after the delivery
- With common use–2%
- With correct and consistent use–0.5%
- Variable effect since 6% ovulate before first menses.

Advantages
- Contraception starts immediately after childbirth
- Encourages the best breastfeeding pattern
- No additional cost
- No appliances/supplies/procedures

Disadvantage
- Difficult for working mothers

WITHDRAWAL METHOD (COITUS INTERRUPTUS)

Ejaculation to be effected outside the vagina by withdrawing the penis just before the ejaculation.

Disadvantages
- Needs a great motivation, self-control or willpower in the male partner.
- Inadequate orgasm
- Female partner may develop sex neurosis, pelvic congestion syndrome with dysmenorrhoea.

Advantages
- Inexpensive
- No medical supervision
- No harm
- Planning for the sexual act not required

Use effectiveness
10–30% failure rate in the first year.

25 Barrier Contraception

These devices act as barriers to prevent the union of sperms and ovum.

Classification

Male barriers: Condoms

Female barriers:
- Spermicides: Creams, jellies, suppositories, foam tablets
- Mechanical barriers
  - Unmedicated
    - ♦ Female condom
    - ♦ Vaginal diaphragm
    - ♦ Cervical caps
  - Medicated: Contraceptive vaginal sponge.

CONDOMS

Condoms are sheaths to cover penis and collect semen during intercourse, thus preventing sperms from entering into the female genital tract.

Condoms are also known as French Letter, prophylactics, protectives and rubber sheaths.

Device

- Made of latex rubber
- Usually available as lubricated

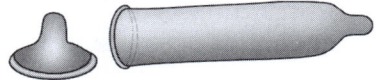

Fig. 25.1: Condom

213

- Cylindrical in shape
- Length 15–20 cm
- Diameter 3–3.5 cm
- Thickness of rubber 0.003–0.007 mm
- Ring of rolled latex rubber at proximal end
- Closed at distal end with a teat for semen collection at the distal end.

Types

a. Regular condoms
  - Teat ended (Fig. 25.1)
  - Plain ended
b. Dry, pre lubricated or Nonoxinol-9 coated spermicidal condom.

Use

Storage in cool dry place protected from sunlight, heat, moisture is necessary to avoid its deterioration.

Condoms are for single use only.

Checking the expiry date and careful opening of the pack necessary.

Rolled condom is placed over the tip of the **erect** penis and unrolled along the shaft. While using teat ended condom, semen collection teat is pinched to expel out air from it. This prevents air trapping and rupture of condom after ejaculation.

If required inert water-based lubricant (K-Y Jelly) may be used. The best lubricant would be spermicidal jelly as it increases the efficacy as well. Any hydrocarbon or oily lubricants like vaseline, creams should not be used since they may damage latex rubber and increase the chance of rupture.

Penis should be withdrawn with condom over it, after the erection subsides. Condom should be removed by rolling it again over the penis. After use, condom should be checked for its integrity before discarding. A knot should be tied at the open end of the condom to avoid spillage. It is safely disposed in dustbins after wrapping in paper, not to be thrown in commodes or flushed in latrines. Can be buried under soil.

Advantages
- No serious drawbacks
- Easily available without medical prescription.
- In India, Nirodh is available free of charge in Government centers and at highly subsidized rate outside. At some places available in vending machines also.
- Harmless device if used with proper precautions.
- Reliable method (failure rate 3%) with proper and consistent use.
- Can prevent STDs including HIV and vaginal infections and their subsequent complications (dual protective method).
- Protects from precancerous lesions and cancer of cervix.
- Helps in prolonging the act of coitus by delaying ejaculation. It can prevent premature ejaculation.

Disadvantages
- Risk of rupturing inside vagina. Reported breakage and slippage rates range between 4 and 13%. This may lead to failure and pregnancy. Emergency contraception should be used within 72 hours of such events.
- May not give so much protection against Herpes genitalis, HPV or diseases which cause sores on skin not covered by condom
- Wearing interferes with sexual act
- May decrease sensation during sexual act
- Every time new condom has to be used
- Woman has to depend on male partner's cooperation
- Some individuals may have allergy to latex who get redness, itching, swelling following use. Immediate washing of the area and topical steroids are helpful. Nonlatex condoms may be used by these individuals.

There is no scientific evidence that N-9-lubricated condoms provide any additional protection against pregnancy or STIs compared with condoms lubricated with other products.

BARRIER DEVICES FOR FEMALES

Though these devices create a physical barrier for sperms in female vagina, they cannot form a watertight partition. Hence, used singly they have got higher failure rate. However, they serve to be good vehicles for spermicidal agents and their combined success rate is fairly high.

FEMALE CONDOM

Device

- Made of polythene sac of 7 cm diameter and 15 cm length.
- Its one end is blind pouch which rests at the vault of vagina. At this end there is a smaller ring which facilitates its insertion. This ring helps retention of female condom inside the vagina and prevents it from falling down.
- The other end having a polyurethane ring lies outside the vagina covering vulva (Fig. 25.2).

Advantages

- Inserted inside well in advance of the sexual act; hence does not affect the libido.
- User dependent, female controlled option
- It provides protection against STD and HIV infection.

Disadvantages

- Requires high motivation
- Intercourse is noisy and slippage may occur
- High failures (5% with correct and consistent use).

Instructions for Use

Never re-use a female condom. Always check expiry date. Take care not to damage with nails when removing from packet. It may be inserted any time before sex.

In a comfortable position, e.g. squatting or one leg up on a chair, hold the closed end of the condom and squeeze the ring

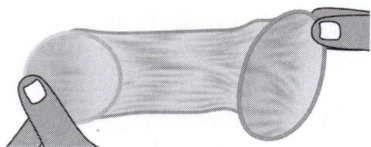

Fig. 25.2: Female condom

between thumb and middle finger. Using the other hand to open the labia, push the ring as high into the vagina as possible. Place the middle finger into the open end of the condom and try to feel the inner ring. Push it high into the vagina. Make sure the outer ring is lying close to the vulva.

It is advisable to guide the penis into the condom, to avoid slipping between condom and vagina. To remove the condom, twist the outer ring (to trap semen inside) and pull gently.

VAGINAL DIAPHRAGM (DUTCH CAP)

Diaphragms are thin, dome-shaped devices made of latex or silicone and range in size between 55 and 100 mm. The outer rim contains a metal spring (Fig. 25.3).

Diaphragms should lie diagonally between the posterior fornix and behind the pubic bone.

Method of Insertion

1. Size of diaphragm is decided by per vaginal examination. Distance from introitus to highest point in the posterior fornix is usually taken as the diameter of diaphragm.
2. Diaphragm should be inserted prior to coitus and should be retained in vagina at least 6 hours after intercourse.
3. Rim of diaphragm is pressed between thumb and finger to make it oval and inserted in vagina in such a fashion that the convexity of the dome faces posteriorly.
4. When inner margin of the rim has reached in the posterior fornix, its outer end is lifted and pushed inside the vagina in anterior fornix to fit behind the pubic symphysis.
5. The edges are palpated to confirm that the cervix is covered by the device.

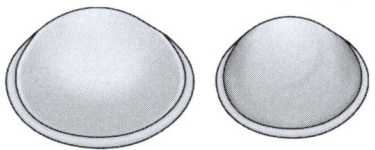

Fig. 25.3: Diaphragm

Advantages
- Safe and economical
- Can be retained inside the vagina for 24 hours
- Can be used repeatedly
- User dependent

Disadvantages
- Needs training for insertion and removal
- Continued motivation for its use is necessary.
- Not protective against HIV infection
- Not acceptable to women who dislike manipulation of genitalia
- High failure rate (15%) when used alone. Efficiency increases when used with a spermicide.
- Size may change after childbirth, significant weight change or after vaginal surgery.
- Not suitable in cases of genital prolapse
- Chances of urinary tract infection.

CERVICAL CAPS

Caps are smaller than diaphragms and sit directly over the cervix held by suction. Caps made of rubber or silicon. These are of three types and are available in different sizes (Fig. 25.4).
- *Cervical cap or check pessary:* This small device of latex rubber fits over the cervix.

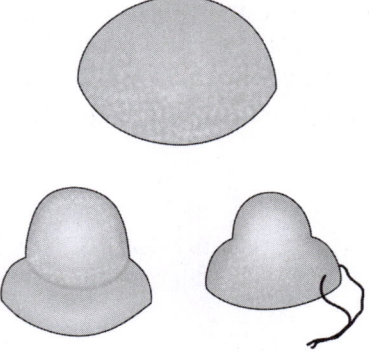

Fig. 25.4: Cervical caps. 1. Vault cap; 2. Check pessary ; 3. Vinule cap

- *Vault cap:* Somewhat vaginal diaphragm shaped, but much smaller sized device is devoid of metal spring
- *Vinule cap:* This is having a flanged base and somewhat elongated dome which increases the degree of suction inside the cap after it is put over the cervix. It is provided with a string for easy removal.

Method of Insertion

1. Like diaphragm, proper size should be ascertained. The device is washed clean before insertion.
2. Cap is filled with 5 ml of spermicidal jelly.
3. It is compressed between thumb and index finger and inserted up to the cervix.
4. The cap is then fitted neatly around the cervix.

Advantages
- Safe and economical
- Can be retained for longer duration (not >48 hours)
- No discomfort during intercourse
- User dependent
- Can be used even in cases with genital prolapse
- Vinule cap having thread can be removed very easily.

Disadvantages
- Medical assistance is required for insertion
- High failure rate (20–30%)
- Chances of infection high (even toxic shock syndrome) if retained for longer period.

Care of Device

After removal, they are to be washed clean with soap and water and stored dry after talc application. Before reuse, the device has to be inspected thoroughly, particularly at the rim edges for wear and tear, in which case the device has to be discarded.

TODAY VAGINAL CONTRACEPTIVE PESSARIES

Active ingredient Nonoxynol-9 (5%)

Mechanism of Action

- Spermicidal
- Soluble foam base immobilizes the sperms by reduction in surface tension.

Method of Use

One pessary to be inserted into the vagina 10 minutes before intercourse. Contraceptive effect lasts for one hour.

Advantages

- Reliable and safe
- Convenient and easy to use
- User dependent

Disadvantages

- Nonoxynol does not offer protection from HIV infection. In fact, it may increase the risk of HIV infection due to genital irritation and ulcers. It does not offer protection against gonnorrhoea or chlamydia. Hence, not recommended for women at high-risk of HIV infection. Some people have reported allergic reactions to Nonoxynol-9
- Low efficacy

CONTRACEPTIVE SPONGE

This device has appearance like vaginal diaphragm, It has a loop for easy removal. Made of polyurethane, it is impregnated with 1 gm Nonoxynol-9 , a spermicidal agent.

Mode of Action

- Nonoxynol-9 acts as spermicidal
- Sponge absorbs the semen
- Device acts as physical barrier also

Method of Insertion

Before insertion, the sponge is soaked in clean water and squeezed of excess water. The device is to be inserted like vaginal diaphragm and must be placed over the cervix to be effective.

The sponge can be inserted up to 24 hours before intercourse. It must be left in place for at least six hours after the intercourse. It should not be left in for more than 30 hours. It has an elastic band to facilitate removal.

Advantages
- Effective for 24 hours irrespective of number of sexual acts
- After insertion, no waiting period

Disadvantages
- May cause allergy/itching, discomfort during coitus, occasional penile itching or sourness after coitus
- Rarely it may cause toxic shock syndrome when left in vagina for longer time.
- Risk of falling in working women
  Failure rate 9–21%
- Not available in India

Does not offer protection against STIs.

26

Hormonal Contraception

Hormones in the hypothalamo-hypophysial-ovarian axis control ovulation. Hence, manipulations of HPO axis by exogenous hormones can inhibit ovulation. This is the main principle of hormonal contraception.

COMBINED ORAL CONTRACEPTIVE PILLS

Oral contraceptive pill is the most effective, safe and reversible method of temporary contraception available at present. Low dose combined oral pills contain less than 0.05 mg of oestrogen.

Types

- *Combined monophasic pills:* All the pills in the pack contain same amount of oestrogen and progestin.
  - Low dose pills–0.03 mg ethinyl estradiol
  - Standard dose pills–0.05 mg ethinyl estradiol
  - Currently pills containing 0.02 mg ethinyl estradiol are available.
  - The progestin component in most pills is Dl Norgestrel or Levonorgestrel. The newer formulations contain Desogestrel, cyproterone acetate, or Drospirenone
  - Desogestrel has less androgen receptor binding. Therefore, it has less androgenic side effects like weight gain, acne, and has favourable lipid profile. However, small risk of venous thromboembolism is observed.
  - Cyproterone acetate is a potent anti androgen
  - Drospirenone is a progestin derived from 17 α-spirono-lactone and has an antimineralocorticoid activity and antiandrogenic activity

- Combined triphasic pills: In the three periods of menstrual cycle, varying amounts of oestrogens and progestogens are used. Initially, the dose of progestogen is low while it is higher in the third phase. Oestrogen dose is increased in the midcycle.

Advantages
- i. *Cycle stability:* Less breakthrough bleeding
- ii. Significant reduction of total dose of hormone per cycle without reducing the efficacy.

Composition of Different Pills

Preparation	Progestogen	Oestrogen
1. Low Dose Pills		
• Mala D	Dl Norgestrel 0.30 mg	EE 0.03 mg
• Ovral L	L Norgestrel 0.15 mg	EE 0.03 mg
• Primovlar 30	L Norgestrel 0.25 mg	EE 0.03 mg
• Novelon	Desogestrel 0.15 mg	EE 0.03 mg
• Femilon	Desogestrel 0.15 mg	EE 0.02 mg
• Lowett	L Norgestrel 0.1 mg	EE 0.02 mg
2. Standard Dose Pills		
• Ovral	Norgestrel 0.25 mg	EE 0.05 mg
• Lyndiol	Lynestrenol 1.0 mg	EE 0.05 mg
3. Triphasic Pill		
• Triquilar		
6 Tabs	Norgestrel 0.050 mg	EE 0.03 mg
5 Tabs	Norgestrel 0.075 mg	EE 0.04 mg
10 Tabs	Norgestrel 0.125 mg	EE 0.03 mg
4. Antiandrogenic Pills		
• Diane 35 +	Cyproterone acetate 2 mg	EE 0.035 mg
• Janya	Drospirenone 3.0 mg	EE 0.03 mg

EE – Ethinyl estradiol
Dl Norgestrel 0.30 mg = L Norgestrel 0.15 mg

Mechanism of Action

1. Inhibition of ovulation by suppressing hypothalamic releasing factors; thereby suppressing FSH and LH release.
2. Affecting implantation by altering maturation of endometrium.

3. Progestogen component reduces the transportation of sperms by making the cervical mucus scanty and viscid.

Selection of Acceptors

Careful selection of acceptors is essential to reduce rare but serious risks associated with pills. Complete history and clinical examination must be carried out to exclude contraindications.

Absolute Contraindications

- Pregnancy
- H/o thromboembolism
- H/o cerebrovascular accident
- Cardiac disease
- Malignancy of breast
- Malignancy of genital tract
- Active liver disease
- H/o cholestatic jaundice during pregnancy
- Migraine

Relative Contraindications

- Undiagnosed abnormal uterine bleeding
- Lactating mothers in first 6 months
- Age over 40 years (over 35 years if smoker)
- Mild hypertension
- Gross obesity
- Diabetes mellitus
- Epilepsy
- Recent history of depression
- Recent history of oligomenorrhoea
- Recent history of amenorrhoea
- H/o jaundice within last 6 months
- Sickle cell disease (trait not a contraindication).

Caution while Oral Contraceptive Use

i. *Drug interaction:* Drugs which may reduce the efficacy of oral contraceptive pills are rifampicin, antibiotics, anticonvulsants and antifungal drugs. Management varies according to the duration of such medication. A back up contraceptive method is recommended for short-term use up to one week. Clients taking such medication for more than one week should be advised to switch over to other contraceptive method.

ii. *Diarrhoea and vomiting:* To avoid failure of pills a back up method such as condom should be used during diarrhoea and/or vomiting and continued for seven days after controlling the symptoms.

iii. *Planned surgery in oral contraceptive user:* Oral contraceptive should be discontinued at least for four weeks prior to contemplated surgery.

Effectiveness and other Advantages

- Highly effective method with failure rate of 0.1% with correct and regular intake by the acceptor
- Safe and reversible
- User dependent
- Privacy not required

Beneficial Effects

1. Reduces the incidence of ectopic pregnancy
2. Menstrual benefits:
   - Relief from menorrhagia, reducing chances of anaemia
   - Relief from dysmenorrhoea
   - Relief from premenstrual tension
   - Regularization of menstrual cycles
3. Reduced incidence of pelvic inflammatory diseases due to thickening of cervical mucus
4. Relief from acne–specially premenstrual type
5. Protection against neoplasia with reduced risk in users
   - Carcinoma endometrium
     - Progesterone inhibits endometrial proliferation
   - Epithelial ovarian cancer
   - Colorectal cancer
   - Benign breast tumours
   - Benign ovarian cysts

6. Marital benefits
   - Not related to sexual act
   - Easy to stop when pregnancy desired

Minor Side Effects

a. Nausea, vomiting
b. Mastalgia
c. Headache
d. Acne
e. Chloasma
f. Depression
g. Breakthrough bleeding is usually due to low oestrogen content in oral contraceptives. Mostly it stops with continued use. Disturbing breakthrough bleeding may be relieved by additional tablet for 2–3 days or changing to preparation containing 50 μg ethinyl estradiol. Switching over to triphasic pill may also be considered. Gynaecological pathology should be excluded before labeling the bleeding as breakthrough bleeding.
h. Mild elevation of blood pressure (which usually disappears on discontinuation of pills).
i. Weight gain: Many of these symptoms disappear on continued use of pills.

Adverse Effects

Major side effects are rare with currently used low dose pills. The reported effects include:

1. Atherosclerotic cardiovascular disease, hypertension and myocardial infarction.

   Progesterone component of the pill increases low-density lipoproteins (LDL) and decreases high density lipoproteins (HDL), thus increasing the risk of atherosclerosis. The oestrogen component has got an opposite effect. As a result, these effects are balanced in currently used low dose pills. The risk factors for cardiovascular complications are:
   - Age >40 years
   - Smoking

- Hypertension
- Diabetes mellitus
- Hyperlipidaemia

2. *Venous thromboembolism:* The oestrogen component of the pill increases the coagulability of blood.
3. *Liver disorder:* Cholestatic jaundice may occur in women having history of cholestatic jaundice during pregnancy.
4. There is increased risk of developing benign liver cell adenoma. However, this is an extremely rare condition.
5. *Carcinogenicity:*
   - *Breast:* Young women do not have appreciably increased risk of breast cancer. Small increase in relative risk of breast cancer in current users which declines with cessation of use (Due to progestogen component that probably result in early detection of existing tumour).
   - *Cervix:* Some studies have shown increased risk of precancerous cervical lesions (CIN) among pill users. The effect of sexual behaviour and smoking has not been considered in these studies.

   It has been shown that use of oral contraceptive pills up to 5 years does not increase the risk of cervical cancer.

   In view of this, all oral contraceptive users should have periodic speculum examination and cervical cytology wherever possible.
   - *Liver:* Long-term oral contraceptive use may be associated with liver cancer, which is an extremely rare cancer.
6. Postpill amenorrhoea is usually seen in women with previous history of infrequent periods. If amenorrhoea continues for two or more cycles, oral contraceptive pills should be discontinued.

   Before diagnosing postpill amenorrhoea, it is necessary to:
   - Enquire about regularity of intake
   - Exclude pregnancy

Other Effects

i. *Return of menstruation and fertility:* No evidence of decreased fertility in oral contraceptive users.

ii. *Pregnancy outcome:* If pregnancy has occurred during pill use or if woman inadvertently continues to consume pills after missing her period for a short period, no significant increased risk of foetal malformation has been observed.

iii. Pills do not offer any protection from HIV or STIs. No clear association between pill use and HIV infection has been identified. Some antiretroviral medicines have drug interactions.

When to Start Pills?

i. Day 5 of menstruation: Pills are effective after 7 days if started on day 5; hence back up contraception is advised for first 7 days. Therefore, it is advised to start the pills from day 1 of the cycle. Breakthrough bleeding is more in first cycle if started on first day.

ii. Day 1 of MTP/spontaneous abortion

iii. After delivery:
- Breastfeeding child: After 6 months
- Non-breastfeeding: After 6 weeks

How to Take the Pill?

1. The first course should be started ideally on first day of the cycle but not later than the fifth day of menstrual cycle by taking the pill marked as start from the pack.
2. For subsequent days, one pill a day should be taken from the pack in the order indicated by the arrows; till all the pills in that pack are over.
3. The pill should be taken everyday at the fixed time, preferably at bedtime.
4. The next pack should be started the very next day if 28 tablets pack is being used. If she is taking 21 tablets preparation, the next pack should be started 7 days after the last tablet of previous pack.

If a Pill is Missed

If a woman misses a pill on a particular night, the missed pill should be taken the next day as soon as she remembers. She should take another pill at night as usual. If she misses 2–3 pills, she should continue taking pills regularly but in addition, she should also use another contraceptive method like condoms till the next menstruation.

Missed Pill

Seven days of uninterrupted pill intake is necessary for adequate suppression of HPO axis. Pill free interval of > 7 days is associated with increased risk of pregnancy.

Missing pills during first, second or third week will have different risk of failure and hence would need different management.

Unprotected sex in preceding 7 days of missing the pill in first week will need medical consultation. If there is no unprotected sex within preceding 7 days of missed pill, a back up method should be used for 7 days and continue taking pills.

Emergency contraception can be used to avoid unintended pregnancy.

Duration of Use

In India continuous use of oral contraceptive pills is recommended up to 5 years. There is no need for periodic withdrawal. However, in women who are otherwise well, low dose oral contraceptive may be continued for several years under medical supervision. For the women who are over 40 years of age, oral contraceptives may be prescribed with caution. Pills containing 0.02 mg ethinyl estradiol may be preferred in such women.

Medical Check up for Oral Contraceptive Users

1. *First:* Before starting the pills
2. *Subsequent:* Yearly
   - Weight
   - Blood pressure
   - Breast palpation
   - Per abdominal examination–liver
   - Per speculum and per vaginal examination.

- Cervical smear
- Urine examination for albumin and sugar.

Warning Signals

ACHES

- **A**bdominal pain
- **C**hest pain
- **H**eadache
- **E**ye problems
- **S**welling of legs

Non-contraceptive Uses of OC Pills

- Treatment of menorrhagia due to anovular DUB
- Primary (spasmodic) dysmenorrhoea when antispasmodics and antiprostaglandins have failed to give relief
- Endometriosis
- Hirsutism
- Polycystic ovarian syndrome (PCOS) when conception is not desired.

A special pill , Diane 35 which contains *Cyproterone acetate* 2 mg + EE 0.035 mg, 21 tablets, is recommended for women with acne, hirsutism. It maintains good cycle control. Cyproterone acetate is a potent anti androgen. It is expensive.

Janya, is another pill prescribed for PCOS which contains *Drospirenone* 3.0 mg + ethinyl estradiol 0.03 mg. Drospirenone is a progestin derived from 17-α-spironolactone and has an antimineralocorticoid and antiandrogenic activity . These pills are devoid of side effects like acne, bloating, weight gain and hypertension.

Oral contraceptive pills should not be used for postmeno-pausal HRT.

Progestogen Only Pills: Mini Pills

Desogestrel 75 mcg daily **(Cerazette):** Continuous regimen (no pill free interval)

Mode of Action

- Ovulation inhibition in 97%
- Thickening of cervical mucus to reduce sperm penetration
- Peak effect within 4 hrs, lasts for 24 hrs

Advantages

- Can be used by lactating mothers and women having contraindications for estrogen containing pills.
- In comparison to Levonorgestrel 30 mcg, lower androgenecity, highly selective, higher rates of inhibition of ovulation. As a result, less chances of having ectopic pregnancy
- Lesser androgenic side effect
- 12 hrs delay need not be considered as missed pill, with LNG mini pill delay should not be more than 3 hrs.

Disadvantages

- Expensive
- No scheduled withdrawl bleedings, no cycles recognizable.

INJECTABLE CONTRACEPTION PROGESTIN ONLY INJECTABLES

- Depot medroxyprogesterone acetate (DMPA) 150 mg every 3 months deep IM
- Norethisterone enanthate (NET-EN) 200 mg every 2 months deep IM

Time of Injection

- Within 7 days of menstruation
- Soon after abortion
- 6 weeks postpartum in breastfeeding women
  Reinjection can be given up to 2 weeks before or after scheduled date.

Mechanism of Action

- Inhibition of ovulation
- Cervical mucus: Thickened and scanty
- Endometrial suppression
- Hindering ovum transport

Side Effects

- Irregular vaginal bleeding, spotting, oligomenorrhoea, amenorrhoea, heavy bleeding in some cases
- Weight gain, headache, dizziness.

Contraindications

- Pregnancy
- Carcinoma of breast or genital tract
- Abnormal uterine bleeding
- Diabetes mellitus
- Stroke
- Coronary artery disease
- Acute liver disease
- Severe hypertension
- Focal migraine
- Liver tumours

Contraceptive Benefits

- Highly effective–0.3 pregnancies/100 women during first year of use
- Rapidly effective
- No effect on lactation and subsequent development of infants.

Non-contraceptive Benefits

- Reduction in menstrual blood loss
- Relief from endometriosis
- Reduced incidence of pelvic inflammatory disease
- Protection against endometrial cancer.

Advantages

- Can be used by women receiving anti-epileptic drugs
- Can be used in women having sickle cell disease.

Disadvantages

- High incidence of menstrual abnormalities
- Delayed return of fertility (average 9 months)

- Acceleration of the growth of existing breast tumours if any (enhanced detection rather than true increase in incidence of breast tumours).

ESTROGEN + PROGESTIN COMBINED INJECTABLES

Not available in India currently
- Cyclofem: DMPA 25 mg + estradiol cypionate 5 mg
- Mesigyna: NET-EN 50 mg + estradiol valerate 5 mg

Administration

- Fisrt injection within 7 days of menstruation
- Re-injection every 30 days ± 3 days

Advantage

Less problems with menstrual cycles as compared to progestin only injectables.

Contraindications

Same as combined pills.

CONTRACEPTIVE VAGINAL RING (NUVARING)

- Once a month contraceptive.
- 3 weeks of continuous use followed by one week of ring free period
- Flexible soft transparent ring, 54 mm in diameter, 4 mm thickness. Contains ethinyl estradiol and etonogestrel
- Provides controlled release of hormones, releases 15 mcg of EE and 120 mcg ENG daily
- Mechanism of action:
  - Inhibition of ovulation
  - Endometrial atrophy
  - Thickenning of cervical mucus

Advantages

- Rapidly reversible
- Highly effective
- Self insertion and removal possible

Disadvantage

Very expensive

CONTRACEPTIVE IMPLANTS

The contraceptive implant is made up of one or more small devices containing progestins that are implanted under the skin of the upper arm under a local anaesthetic. It takes only few minutes to insert the device. These are currently not available in India.

Types of Implants

Norplant 1: A long acting reversible system of progesterone contraception, which consists of 6 non biodegradable sialastic capsules. Each capsule is of 3.4 cm in length having 2.4 mm diameter and contains 36 mg of Levonorgestrel. A set of 6 capsules is placed subdermally in upper part of arm, under local anaesthesia; during days 1 to 7 of menstrual cycle. Effect lasts for 5 years. During first year 50–80 µg Norgestrel is released everyday while subsequently the daily release drops to 30–50 µg.

Implanon: A single-rod implant, 4 cm long and 2 mm in diameter. It consists of 68 mg of Etonogestrel in an ethylene vinyl acetate copolymer core, effective for 3 years.

Etonogestrel is biologically active metabolite of Desogestrel and is significantly more potent than Levonorgestrel.

- Inserted in medial aspect of left arm, 8–10 cm above medial epicondyle
- *Time of insertion:* Day 1 to 5 of menstrual period, immediately following first trimester MTP, 21–28 days following delivery
- *Efficacy:* 0.3 to 1.1 pregnancies/HWY in first year of use
- Higher frequency of amenorrhea and oligomenorrhea
- Decrease in the frequency of adverse effects such as weight gain, headache, and acne
- When the rod is removed, the return to fertility is rapid, with the return of ovulation within 3 weeks
- May be less effective in overweight women.

Mode of Action

- Suppressing ovulation

- Reducing sperm permeability of cervical mucus by increasing its viscosity and by changing its composition
- Inhibiting implantation by suppressing endometrial growth.

Advantages
- Highly effective long acting method
- Reversible soon after removal
- No oestrogenic side effects
- It does not affect lactation adversely.
- No aftercare required
- No interference in sexual life.

Disadvantages
- Medical personnel required for insertion and removal
- Initially expensive
- May cause irregular spotting or oligomenorrhoea.
- Increased incidence of ectopic pregnancies in cases of failure
- May cause transient ovarian cysts
- At times removal may be difficult
- Infection/haematoma during insertion or removal
- Rarely devices may get expelled out.

Contraceptive Patch

This transdermal patch contains combination of ethinyl estradiol (EE) and progestin norgestimate (NGM). It delivers each hormone continuously at a steady rate for 7 days with an average dose of 25 µg of EE and 250 µg of NGM per day.

The patch is applied immediately after the menstrual period is over. Each patch is worn for 7 days continuously which is then replaced by another patch. Such 3 patches are used successively after which there is a 7 days *patch free* interval.

EMERGENCY CONTRACEPTION

Women who have experienced unprotected sex like breakage of barrier, failure to use planned method, missed pills for 3 days or sexual assault can protect themselves from pregnancy by using emergency contraception.

Methods

1. *Progestogen:* Levonorgestrel 1.5 mg single dose as early as possible within 72 hours of unprotected sex prevents 85% of pregnancies. Can be taken up to 120 hours but its efficacy is reduced. It has less side effects than Yuzpe method.

2. *Oestrogen/progesteron combination (Yuzpe regimen):* 0.1 mg ethinyl estradiol + 0.5 mg Levonorgestrel (LNG) pills; 2 pills given at 12 hourly interval within 72 hours of unprotected sex.
   Side effects: Nausea, vomiting, tiredness, dizziness.
   Prevents 75% of pregnancies.

3. *Mifepristone (RU486):* Single dose of 600 mg has good efficacy and almost no gastrointestinal side effects, however, menstrual disturbances occur commonly. WHO studies have shown that lower doses of Mifepristone (10 mg and 50 mg) have similar efficacy and lesser problem of menstrual delay. These hormonal methods of emergency contraception are effective for single coital exposure during that cycle.

4. *Intrauterine device:* Insertion of IUD within 5 days of intercourse gives protection against pregnancy; further it gives a continued regular contraception.

Mode of Action

- Asynchronization of ovum transport and endometrial development; interfering with implantation.
- Interference with development of corpus luteum; hence no postovulatory progesterone. This leads to fall in the levels of carbonic anhydrase (CAH) which is responsible for stickiness of the blastocyst.
- Progestogens increase the intrauterine pH which immobilize the sperms.
- IUDs directly interfere with implantation: Copper in IUD has direct embryotoxic action.

Risks of Emergency Contraception

Emergency contraception does not increase the risk of ectopic pregnancy. Also it does not increase the risk of terratogenicity in case of its failure or if mistakenly taken in early pregnancy. Pregnancy rates of different methods are shown in Table 26.1.

Table 26.1: Pregnancy rate with emergency contraception

Method	Pregnancy rate
• Single coital exposure anytime of cycle	8%
• Midcycle exposure	20–50%
• Yuzpe regimen	2–3%
• Mifepristone (600 mg)	0%
• LNG	1.2%
• Cu-T	0.1–0.2%

NON-STEROIDAL ORAL PILL: CENTCHROMAN

This type of contraceptive pill is developed in India.
• Weekly, non-steroidal pill
• Effective within a week
• Weak oestrogenic and potent antioestrogenic properties, selective estrogen receptor modulator
• Also shown to be beneficial for treating dysfunctional uterine bleeding, osteoporosis and premenstrual syndrome.

Mechanism of Action

Anti-implantation effect by creating asynchrony between the developing zygote and endometrial maturation.

Available Preparations

Saheli, Sevista
Dose: 30 mg biweekly for 3 months; weekly thereafter. Start the tablet on day 1 of the period.

Advantages
• No effect on endocrine system
• No side effects
• Reversible

Disadvantages
• Prolonged menstrual cycles (>45 days)
• Cystic enlargement of ovaries
• High failure rates observed (typical use 9%, correct use around 2%).

27

Intrauterine Contraceptive Devices

Classification

1. *First generation devices:* Inert nonmedicated devices, e.g. Grafenberg's ring, Ota ring, Lippes loop.
2. *Second generation devices:* Medicated devices in which metals like copper, zinc and silver are used, e.g. CuT 200, multiload, CuT 380 Ag.
3. *Third generation devices:* Newer medicated devices in which hormones (progesterone, levonorgestrel) or antifibrinolytic agents (epsilon aminocaproic acid, tranexamic acid) are incorporated.

SOME CURRENTLY USED DEVICES

1. CuT 380 A (Fig. 27.1)

- T-shaped polyethylene frame with 380 sq mm of copper
- 176 mg of copper wire around verticle stem
- 66.5 mg copper sleeve on each transverse arm

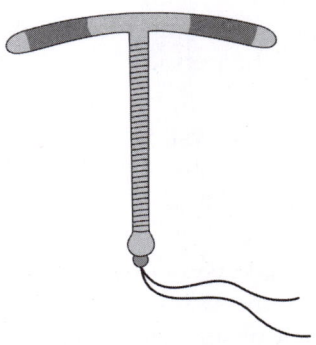

Fig. 27.1: CuT 380 A

- Frame contains barium sulfate for radiologic visualization
- Length 36 mm/Width 32 mm
- Tip of vertical arm–a bulb of 3 mm in diameter
- Polyethylene monofilament tied through the bulb for detection and removal
- High efficacy–>99%
- Effective life–10 years
- Available free in national family welfare program.

2. Multiload Cu 250 and Cu 375 (Fig. 27.2)

- Made of polypropylene with barium sulfate incorporated
- Available as multiload Cu 250 having 250 sq mm copper wire wound around the vertical limb and Cu 375 having 375 sq mm copper wire
- Effective life is 3 years for Cu 250 and 5 years for Cu 375
- Shield shaped
- Flexible spiculed plastic arms help it to be retained in the uterine cavity without stretching it.
- Special inserter of withdrawal type without a plunger.

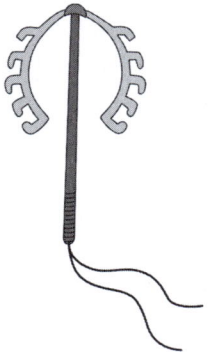

Fig. 27.2: Multiload

3. Copper-T 200 (Fig. 27.3)

- T-shaped device made of polyethylene with barium sulfate incorporated in it for radio-opacity.
- 200 sq mm copper wire is wound round the vertical stem.

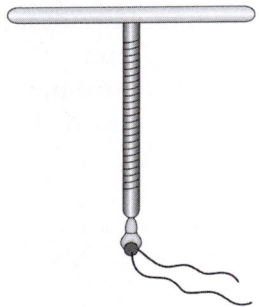

Fig. 27.3: CuT 200

- Two nylon threads at the lower end of the vertical stem.
- Inserter is of withdrawal type containing an outer tube and an inner plunger; an adjustable guard is provided on the tube.
- Effective life is 3 years.
- First copper bearing IUD in national family welfare program.

4. Mirena Intrauterine System (Fig. 27.4)
- Levonorgestrel releasing IUD
- 20 µg Levonorgestrel released per day
- Effective life–5 years
- Failure rate 0.1%– 0.4%
- Very expensive

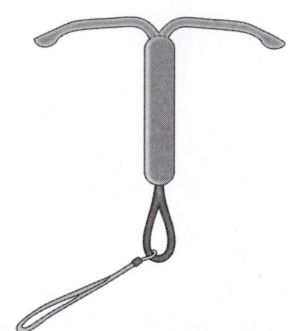

Fig. 27.4: Mirena

- Special insertion technique as per manufacturer's instructions
- Can be used for treatment of idiopathic menorrhagia and endometrial hyperplasia.

Mechanism of Action

Precise mechanism of action of these IUDs is not known. However, following theories have been postulated:

1. IUD stimulates an inflammatory or foreign body response in the uterine cavity resulting in cellular and biochemical changes in the endometrium and uterine fluid, creating a hostile atmosphere for the sperms and the fertilized ovum. Foreign body giant cells, mononuclear cells, plasma cells and macrophages appearing in the endometrium engulf, the spermatozoa or the fertilized ovum by phagocytosis. Macrophages produce prostaglandins, which lead to asynchronous development of endometrium and increased uterine activity.

2. Because of the inflammatory changes in the endometrium the normal cycle gets delayed and the endometrium becomes inhospitable to implantation of the fertilized embryo.

3. Copper interferes with the enzymes in the uterine cavity. Copper increases inflammatory reaction and increases myometrial contractions to prevent the implantation. Copper alters the biochemical composition of the cervical mucus to have adverse effect on sperm motility, capacitation and survival.

4. Progesterone releasing IUDs maintain high progesterone and relatively low oestrogen levels in the uterus. Thus the endometrium in the progesterone phase does not allow implantation. Small amount of progesterone released by these devices does not affect the ovarian function.

Advantages

a. Highly effective
b. Longer duration of use and effectivity
c. Completely reversible on removal of the device
d. No systemic effects

e. Recurrent motivation not required
f. Inexpensive for the patient
g. Does not interfere with coital act
h. No effect on lactation

Selection of Case

a. Complete history, menstrual and sexual risk behavior
b. Complete physical examination including gynaecological examination
c. Cytological smear from cervix
d. All the contraindications are ruled out.
e. Woman should be well motivated.
f. Written consent in a prescribed form.

WHO medical eligibility criteria for IUD describe four categories for eligibility depending upon the conditions present.

- Category 1: No restriction for use
- Category 2: Can generally use IUD (advantages outweigh the risks, however, additional care required)
- Category 3: IUD not recommended (risks outweigh the advantages)
- Category 4: Unacceptable risks, should not use IUD.

Contraindications

a. Known or suspected pregnancy
b. Pelvic infection–current or within six weeks in immediate past
c. Pelvic tuberculosis
d. Having high-risk of gonorrhea, chlamydia having purulent cervical discharge
e. Menorrhagia, severe dysmenorrhoea
f. Undiagnosed genital bleeding
g. Suspected malignancy of the genital tract
h. During follow-up for gestational trophoblastic disease
i. Congenital uterine abnormalities or uterine fibroids distorting uterine cavity that interfere with insertion or prevent proper placement of IUD.

Category 2 Conditions

- Age <20 years, nullipara
- Soon after second trimester abortion, <48 hours postpartum
- HIV infected, AIDS on ARV therapy if clinically well
- Risk of STI other that gonorrhea, chlamydia
- Valvular heart disease (prophylactic antibiotics advised)
- Anemia (nutritional supplements advised)
- Cervical stenosis

Time of Insertion

1. *Interval insertion:* This is usually carried out in the post-menstrual phase of the cycle, preferably on 4th or 5th day, for the following reasons:
   - Pregnancy is ruled out.
   - Cervix is somewhat softer and patulous.
   - Insertion is easy and safe.
   - Postinsertion bleeding is less noticeable in last few days of menstruation.

   However, for a woman who is reasonably sure that she is not pregnant, the best time for IUD insertion is when she comes to the health centre with a request for IUD insertion.

2. *Postpartum insertion:* Most ideal time for IUD insertion in postpartum period is six weeks after delivery (anytime beyond 4 weeks). Can be inserted <48 hours postpartum by a trained provider if there is no evidence of infection. However, there is higher chance of expulsion.

3. *Postabortal insertion:* IUD can be inserted immediately after first trimester spontaneous or induced abortion. IUD inserted immediately after second trimester abortions, carry five times more chances of expulsion than immediately after first trimester abortions.

4. *Postcoital insertion:* IUD inserted within five days after an unprotected intercourse can give protection from pregnancy by interfering with the implantation of the fertilized ovum in the uterus. Advantage of postcoital CuT insertion is that it provides an effective continuous method of contraception.

Instruments

- Sim's speculum with anterior vaginal wall retractor
- Volsellum
- Uterine sound
- Sponge holding forceps
- Scissors
- IUD with its respective inserter.

Sterilization of IUD and Inserter

Copper IUDs and their inserters are available in gamma ray presterilized packets.

Methods of Insertion

1. First, a careful bimanual examination is carried out to note the position, size and regularity of uterus
2. Cervix is visualized.
3. Anterior lip of cervix is grasped by volsellum and slight traction is given on it to straighten the uterocervical canal.
4. The cervix is cleaned with a piece of gauze soaked in antiseptic lotion.
5. The length and direction of the uterine cavity is determined with the help of uterine sound and the blue collar is adjusted, accordingly.
6. The device is loaded in the inserter tube and inserted in the uterine cavity. The thread peeping into vagina is trimmed at about 2–3 cm distance from the external os of cervix.

There are different techniques of insertion:

Withdrawal technique is used for insertion of CuT. The tube of inserter bearing the device is introduced right up to the fundus of the uterus. The device in it is fixed by fixing the plunger by thumb. The outer tube is then withdrawn while the plunger maintains the IUD in proper position in the uterine cavity. Then the plunger is withdrawn with the outer tube.

Advantages of withdrawal technique

- Proper placement of CuT high up at the uterine fundus is possible (Fig. 27.5)

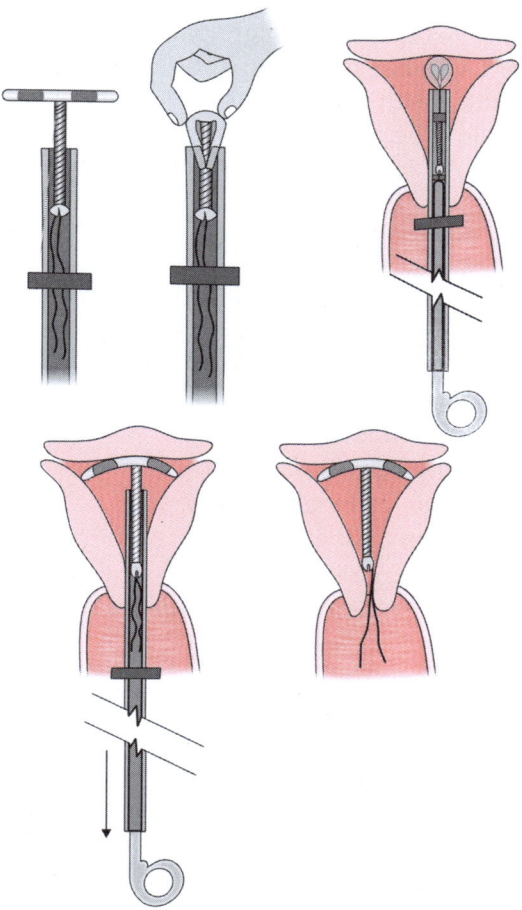

Fig. 27.5: CuT 380 A insertion

- Risk of fundal perforation is less
- Chances of expulsion of the device are less.

Multiload Cu 250 does not require plunger. The tube containing the device is introduced into the uterine cavity up to the fundus of the uterus and then just withdrawn. The spikes of the arched arms hold on the uterine cavity.

Post Insertion Instructions

1. Common side effects, viz. slight pain in the lower abdomen and slight vaginal bleeding, should be explained to the patient with assurance.
2. Patient should be familiarized with the type of IUD and its active life. Accordingly, she should be advised to get it changed.
3. Check the threads regularly and report for follow-up in case they are not felt.
4. Inspect all the pads and tampons during menstrual period, particularly in first three months for expulsion of the device.
5. Report to the physician immediately if:
   - Threads are not felt in the vagina
   - Device is expelled out
   - Period is missed
   - Unusually heavy bleeding occurs
   - Severe pain in abdomen
   - Vaginal discharge with fever
6. She should be explained the schedule of follow-up.

Follow-up

During the visits, complaints if any are noted and managed.

First Visit–after One Month of Insertion

- Mild pain and bleeding—assurance and analgesics
- Severe pain due to pelvic infection—antibiotics
  - If no response within 48 hours then removal of device
- Heavy bleeding—hormones, antiprostaglandins
  - If continuous uncontrolled bleeding, then device is removed.
- Thread is checked per vaginum.

Second Visit–after Three Months

- The amount of bleeding and pain during menstrual periods is noted.
- Thread is checked per vaginum.

Subsequent Visits

Six monthly, preferably for first year and then annually for subsequent one to two years till the device is changed or removed.

When Threads Not Seen or Felt

If threads are not felt by the patient in the vagina, then she should see the physician immediately. In such cases, physician should look for the threads by speculum examination. If the threads are not seen, then action is to be taken according to the Flow chart 27.1.

Complications

1. *Bleeding:* Increased amount of bleeding often accompanied by pain is the commonest complication resulting in removal of IUD in 5–15% of women. Bleeding can be of three types
   - Excessive menstrual blood loss

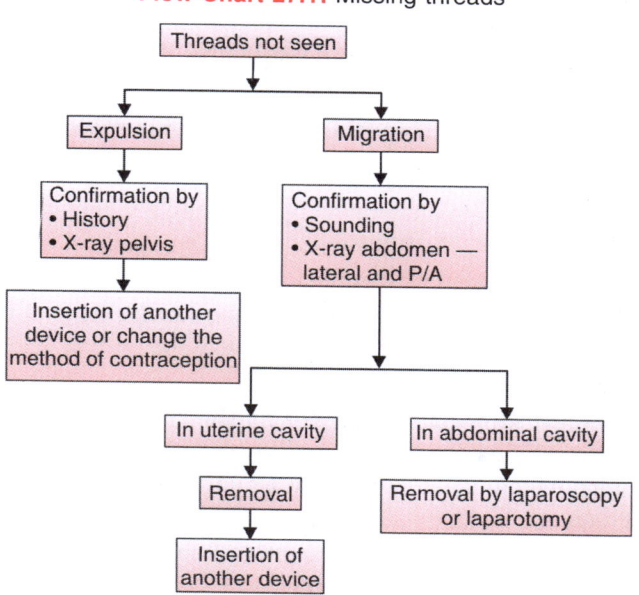

Flow Chart 27.1: Missing threads

- Longer duration of menstrual bleeding
- Intermenstrual bleeding

Management

- Slight intermenstrual bleeding due to mechanical irritation of the endometrium stops as the healing takes place over the time.
- Premenstrual spotting for few days usually needs only reassurance and acceptance.
- Response to oral contraceptive pills, coagulant drugs, vitamins, etc. is usually unsatisfactory in controlling the bleeding. Many drugs are being tried:
  - Non-steriodal antiinflammatory drugs like prostaglandin synthetase inhibitors, e.g. indomethacin, naproxen, mefenamic acid, etc. are tried with success
  - IUDs releasing antifibrinolytic agents like EACA and Tranexamic acid are being tried.

2. *Infection:* Infection can occur in two ways:
   - Failure to observe proper aseptic precautions
   - Exacerbation of preexisting subclinical infection
   - New STI

Most infections occur within 20 days of insertion.

Prevention

- Proper aseptic technique
- Proper selection of cases
- Using devices having monofilament tails.

Treatment

Treatment should be started at the earliest by prompt diagnosis by early symptoms like abdominal pain, adnexal tenderness, painful cervical manipulations, fever and vaginal discharge.

Use of broad spectrum antibiotics for 48 hours following which the IUD should be removed.

3. Pregnancy
   - The chance of pregnancy as a result of IUD failure is less than 1% with modern IUDs. The consequences of pregnancy with IUD in situ are as follows:
     - About 50% of the pregnancies abort spontaneously. Usually abortion occurs in second trimester. Abortion is often complicated by sepsis. Hence the risk to life and health is considerably greater.
     - Risk of preterm deliveries, stillbirths and low birth weight is considerably increased.
     - There is no evidence of birth defects in such pregnancies.

Management
   - Early diagnosis should be made soon after missing a period.
   - If the thread is seen, the device should be removed. MTP is advised considering the risks in continuing the pregnancy. If the patient wants that pregnancy, it may be continued.
   - If the thread is not seen, no attempt should be made to confirm the presence of device in the uterine cavity. The patient should be explained the risk of continuing pregnancy and MTP should be advised.
     - If the patient wishes to continue her pregnancy inspite of knowing the risks, then she should have frequent antenatal check up and her delivery should be supervised. Usually, the device is recovered after the third stage.
   - Ectopic pregnancy cannot be prevented by IUD. IUD gives protection only against uterine pregnancy. IUD does not increase the risk of ectopic pregnancy. However, when pregnancy occurs in an IUD user, it is more likely to be ectopic than intrauterine. Therefore, if an IUD user reports with missed period, with or without pelvic pain possibility of ectopic pregnancy should always be kept in mind.
   - Women already at a higher risk of ectopic pregnancy, e.g. previous pelvic inflammatory disease, ectopic pregnancy, tubal surgery, preferably should avoid an IUD insertion.

4. *Uterine perforation:* Perforation is rare and occurs mostly at the time of insertion. The factors include:
   - Less experienced persons
   - Push-out technique
   - Improper technique–failure to stabilize the uterus or assess the length and direction of the uterus before insertion.
   - Postpartum period–when the uterus is soft.
   - Uterus is acutely anteflexed or retroflexed.

Diagnosis

- Patient may complain of pain in abdomen and inability to feel the thread.
- On examination the thread is not seen in the vagina.
- Patient has not noticed expulsion.

Confirmation

- Ultrasonography
- P/A and lateral views of X-ray with sound in the uterine cavity.

Management

Copper IUDs initiate inflammation and adhesions in the peritoneal cavity. Hence, they must be removed. Open, linear and nonmedicated devices can be left alone, or removed as per patient's wish.

Removal of migrated IUD can be undertaken by laparotomy or laparoscopy. Usually, due to adhesions with omentum, laparoscopic removal of copper IUD may be difficult and laparotomy may be required.

Some other suitable method of contraception should be advised for further contraception. If the patient has completed her family, tubectomy may be performed simultaneously while removing the migrated IUD.

5. *Expulsion:* Chances of expulsion are high in:
   - Immediate postpartum or insertion following second trimester abortion as the uterus is contracting and involuting.

- *Faulty technique:* If IUD is not placed high enough in the uterine cavity or IUD remains deformed in the inserter for more than 3–5 minutes.
- *Device:* Smaller sized devices carry more risk of getting expelled out. Type of the device also plays an important role. Lippes loop had a higher expulsion rate than copper device.
- *Parity:* More chances of expulsion in nullipara
- *Age:* Expulsion rate declines with the age.
- *Period:* Expulsion generally occurs during the first three months of insertion and usually during menstrual period.

If expulsion is noticed then another device, preferably of larger size should be introduced. If the device gets expelled out even after second insertion, then the woman should be advised to change the method of contraception. If expulsion goes unnoticed, unwanted pregnancy may follow.

6. *Migration of the device within the uterine cavity*
   - The device may somersault.
   - The device may get embedded into the uterine wall (incomplete perforation).
   - Thread may get pulled into the uterine cavity.

In such cases, thread is not seen at the follow-up examination. USG or uterine sounding and X-rays reveal its position. Such device should be removed, as it is difficult to follow the patient. Hysteroscopy makes removal of the device possible under vision. After removal another device can be introduced if the patient wishes so, otherwise another method of contraception is advised.

7. *Pain:* Mild colicky pain in hypogastric region few days after the insertion does not need any treatment. Severe pain may be due to:
   - Pelvic infection
   - Ectopic pregnancy
   - Uterine perforation
   - Intrauterine pregnancy in the process of abortion

Indications for Removal of IUD

1. Pelvic infection not responding to antibiotics
2. Profuse bleeding
3. Partial expulsion
4. Embedded device–migration of the device into the uterine wall with thread pulled up
5. Pregnancy
6. After effective life of the IUD is over
7. Perforation
8. Uterine or cervical malignancy.

Method of Removal

- Visualization of cervix
- The tail of IUD is grasped with artery forceps.
- Traction is applied and the device is removed.

Difficulties

- If removal is difficult by above method, then cervicouterine canal is steadied and straightened with volsellum and then the threads are pulled to remove the IUD.
- If threads are not visible, hysteroscopy helps in locating the device in the uterine cavity and also in easy removal.
- Shirodkar's hook (Fig. 27.6) or some other grasping instrument like artery forceps can be introduced into the uterine cavity to remove the device.
- At times, dilatation and curettage or aspiration of the uterine cavity by suction curette may be useful in retrieving threads that are retracted into the uterine cavity.

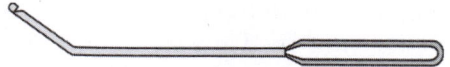

Fig. 27.6: Shirodkar's hook

28 | Female Sterilization

Indications

1. For family limitation on socioeconomic grounds
2. For medical reasons like heart disease, renal disease, multiple caesarean sections, etc.
3. Eugenic grounds–mentally retarded patient.

Timing for Surgery

- Puerperal
- Postabortal
- Interval
- Concurrent with other surgical procedures like caesarean section, MTP, prolapse repair, etc.

Puerperal Tubectomy

On the first day of delivery, the patient is exhausted due to the stress of the delivery. Also it is always advised to observe the patient for primary postpartum haemorrhage. Hence, she is taken for tubectomy after 48 hours of delivery.

Advantages

a. During this period, the uterus is an abdominal organ and hence the operation is technically easy and can be performed under local anaesthesia.
b. It is very convenient for the patient and her family as mostly for the first ten days she is already in the hospital. Also the newborn is with her and additional help is already sought by the family.
c. Motivation of the patient for sterilization is easy.

Interval Tubectomy

It should be performed within 7–10 days of last menstrual period, i.e. preovulatory phase of the cycle. If operated during the postovulatory phase of the cycle, there is a chance of operating after the conception.

Eligibility

- Married
- Age: Between 22 and 45 years
- Having at least one living child elder than 1 year
- Children healthy and well immunized.

Contraindications

No permanent contraindication. However the procedure should be delayed until the medical conditions are treated and resolved.

Women having conditions that increase the anesthetic risk or surgical difficulties and risk should be referred to well equipped center.

Counseling Points

- Information about all the available methods of family planning. Couple should be encouraged to make an informed decision of sterilization voluntarily
- Safe and simple procedure
- Permanent method of contraception
- Surgical procedure with small risk of complications requiring further treatment
- Little chance of failure (0.1%–0.5%). In case of failure, the resulting pregnancy can be terminated by MTP
- Surgery for reversal is possible but involves a major surgery and its success cannot be guaranteed.

Informed Consent

- Consent obtained when the person is not under any physical or mental stress and not sedated
- Without any coercion

- Offering full information about the procedure
- Patient's own written consent on a prescribed form
- Written consent of the spouse not required
- For mentally ill patients, consent by the legal guardian/ spouse is obtained after having mental illness certified by a psychiatrist.

Medical Fitness

- Haemoglobin >= 8.0 gm%
- Urine analysis: Exclude abnormalities, infection
- Examination and treatment of any skin lesions, especially at the operation site
- Exclude pregnancy
- Exclude pelvic infection, peritonitis, STD
- Exclude acute systemic infections, active liver disease, jaundice, febrile illness
- Review past medical history and perform a complete physical examination to exclude tuberculosis, bronchial asthma, epilepsy, heart disease, hypertension, thyrotoxicosis, psychiatric illness, etc.
- Look for gross obesity or multiple scars of previous laparotomies which may warn about difficulties during the surgery
- Ensure that the patient is fully immunized against tetanus
- Following delivery ensure that the pregnancy complications like puerperal infection, hemorrhage, hypertension, are appropriately treated and have resolved
- Examine the baby for any illness
- In postabortal state, exclude sepsis, severe postabortal hemorrhage.

Preoperative Preparation

- Bath and cleaning the area
- NBM for at least 6 hours prior to surgery
- Simple enema before the surgery
- Premedication given IM 30 minutes before surgery.
  - Inj. Atropine 0.6 mg

      – Inj. Pethidine 50–100 mg or Inj. Pentazocine 30 mg
      – Inj. Promethazine 25 mg

Empty the urinary bladder by voiding urine before entering the operation theatre.

Anaesthesia

- *Local:* Lignocaine 1% (maximum 20 ml) without adrenaline
- Spinal or general anaesthesia given if required

Surgical Technique

- Minilaparotomy
- Laparoscopic tubal occlusion

PUERPERAL TUBECTOMY

Instruments

- General instruments for laparotomy
- Right angled retractor
- Babcock's forceps

Steps

1. Abdomen painted and draped
2. Anaesthesia of choice given
3. Uterine fundus is palpated. Local anaesthesia is infiltrated at the proposed site of incision.
4. Abdomen is opened in layers.
5. Abdominal wall is retracted by right angled retractor.
6. Fallopian tube is visualized and grasped by Babcock's forceps. Its identity is confirmed by tracing it up to the fimbrial end.
7. Site of occlusion should be within 2–3 cm from the uterine cornu in the isthmial portion. It has highest potential of the success of reversal surgery if required in future.
8. Care is taken to avoid damage to the blood vessels, ovaries or surrounding tissue.
9. Excision of 1 cm segment of the tube is done. The open ends of the cut tube are ligated with 1/0 chromic catgut.

10. The tubal stumps are inspected for any bleeding.
11. Abdomen is closed in layers.

Postoperative Care

- Nil by mouth for 6 hours
- Monitor the vital signs
- Prophylactic antibiotics
- Keep the incision area clean and dry
- Stitches removal and wound inspection on the 7th day.

INTERVAL STERILIZATION BY MINILAPAROTOMY

Anaesthesia

Local anaesthesia

Instruments

- All the instruments for laparotomy
- Sim's speculum
- Uterine manipulator

Principle of Surgery

Instead of introducing the instruments in the abdominal cavity to reach the tubes, the tubes are brought to the level of the incision by manipulating and elevating the uterus vaginally.

Steps

1. Patient is made to lie in semilithotomy position.
2. Cervix is visualized.
3. Anterior lip of the cervix is grasped and uterine elevator (volsellum-cum-sound) is introduced through the cervix to elevate the uterus against the anterior abdominal wall.
4. Small transverse suprapubic incision of 3–5 cm length is taken and the abdomen is opened.
5. Due to the elevation of the uterus, the tubes are found under the incision. A loop of each tube is pulled out of the incision, ligated and excised by Pomeroy's method.
6. The stumps are left in and the peritoneum is sutured by a purse string stitch, using catgut. Abdomen is closed in layers.

Postoperative

The patient is observed for 4 hours. She can be discharged on the same day or after removal of stitches.

Prophylactic antibiotics are given.

Advantages
- Safe, quick, and simple procedure
- Does not require hospitalization
- Very few complications
- No need for special equipment or special training
- Economical method
- Suitable for rural areas with limited facilities.

Disadvantages
- Difficult in obese patients
- Difficult in presence of adhesions due to previous infections or surgical procedures.

In cases of puerperal patients, minilaparotomy needs a little modification in the technique. Uterus being an abdominal organ, uterine elevator is not required and the uterus can be moved through the incision with a finger to bring the tubes to the incision.

Complications of Abdominal Tubectomy

Intraoperative

1. *Injury to the intestines or bladder:* Usually occurs while opening the peritoneal cavity.

   Prevention
   - Emptying the bladder by voiding before surgery
   - Opening the peritoneum carefully after inspecting its transparency and palpating it
2. *Bleeding:* It commonly occurs from the stumps if the ligatures are not tied properly or if they silp.
3. *Difficulty in catching the tubes;* particularly in fat or apprehensive women in interval cases or in presence of adhesions. In such cases following steps are helpful:
   - Give general anaesthesia

- Enlarge the incision
- Explore the pelvis carefully
4. *Anaesthetic mishaps*
   - Respiratory depression or arrest
   - Cardiac arrest
   - Convulsions and toxic reactions to lignocaine
5. *Mesosalpingeal haematoma* can result if a blood vessel gets punctured and remains unnoticed.
6. *Injury to ovary*
7. In minilaparotomy uterine elevator can cause *uterine perforation* and bleeding.

Immediate Postoperative Period

a. Wound infection and dehiscence
b. Haematoma in the incision
c. Pelvic infection
d. Paralytic ileus and peritonitis
e. Urinary infection
f. Intraperitoneal bleeding if the stump keeps bleeding.

Delayed

a. *Failure:* Pregnancies after sterilization can occur due to:
   - Sterilization performed in the luteal phase of the cycle while the woman had already conceived
   - Surgical errors: Mistaking round ligament or ovarian ligament for fallopian tubes
   - Spontaneous recanalization or reanastomosis
   - Tuboperitoneal or uteroperitoneal fistula
   - Devices like clips and rings may break during application or may slip off the tube later.

   Incidence of failure depends upon
   - Method
     < *Madleners method—1–2%*
     < *Pomeroys mehod—0.1–0.4%*
   - Time of surgery
     < *More at caesarean section*
     < *More at puerperal than at interval tubectomy*
   - Technical skill of the surgeon

b. Chronic pelvic inflammatory disease
c. Incisional hernia
d. *Ectopic pregnancy:* The incidence of ectopic pregnancy is higher in pregnancies resulting after sterilization.
e. Menorrhagia
f. More incidence of hysterectomy in future.

LAPAROSCOPIC STERILIZATION

Laparoscopic sterilization is preferred for interval sterilization and for performing sterilization along with first trimester abortions (Table 28.1 for comparison with minilaparotomy).

Contraindications

In addition to those mentioned under the contraindications for laparoscopy. This procedure should be avoided in pregnancy and puerperium to avoid injury to the uterus and risk of gas embolism through it. This method should be used only when the uterus is pelvic organ.

Instruments

- Complete set of instruments for laparoscopy
- Second puncture trocar and cannula
- Ring/Clip applicator
  In case of single puncture operating laparoscope these are incorporated in the scope itself and second puncture is not required.
- *Silastic bands or tantalum clips:* These are simple and safe appliances with low morbidity and a high potential for reversibility. The bands carry a lesser risk of failure in comparison to clips. The silastic bands have outer diameter of 3.6 mm and inner diameter of 1 mm with thickness of 2.2 mm.

Anaesthesia

Local anaesthesia with premedication or general anaesthesia.

Steps of Operation

1. Trendlenberg position (not more than 15° inclination).
2. Skin incision and puncture with Veress needle (some surgeons prefer direct trocar entry).
3. Pneumoperitoneum is created slowly–1 litre of air or gas (CO_2 preferred as it gets readily absorbed).
4. Introduction of trocar, angled towards the hollow of the sacrum after lifting the abdominal wall.
5. Introduction of telescope and connecting the light source. Single puncture or double puncture technique can be used
6. Tubal occlusion by Falope rings–about 2–3 cm away from the cornual ends.

   If the tubes are thick, oedematous or fixed, rings are not applied and tubal occlusion performed by conventional technique by laparotomy.
7. Inspection of pelvis to verify that both the tubes are occluded, there is no unusual bleeding and there is no visceral injury.
8. Air inside the peritoneal cavity is removed.
9. The cannula is removed with the trocar in it.

Advantages

- When done under local anaestheia, patient can be discharged within 4–6 hours.
- Less operative trauma and rapid postoperative recovery.
- Subsequent reanastomosis of the tube, if required, gives better success rate since the fallopian tube is not damaged to a great extent and the remaining tube is healthy.
- Suitable for mass sterilization camps.

Disadvantages

- Equipment is extremely costly.
- Prior training and experience in the technique is essential.
- Risk of complications is high.

VAGINAL TUBECTOMY

This procedure was performed for interval tubectomy and for tubectomy along with the first trimester MTP. However, due to the disadvantages and greater morbidity, nowadays this

Table 28.1: Laparoscopic sterilization vs minilaparotomy

Laparoscopic	Minilaparotomy
Unsuitable for postpartum sterilization	Suitable for postpartum sterilization
Can be performed under LA. Very rarely GA is required	Though can be performed under LA, may require GA
Can be discharged on the same day	Hospitalization usually for seven days. Discharging patients after 6–24 hrs also has been a safe practice
Costly equipment is required	No special costly equipment is required
Requires high technical skill	Comparatively less technical skill is required
Smooth and quick convalescence	Prolonged convalescence
Complications if met with, are of serious nature, which sometimes may be life-threatening, e.g. air embolism, massive internal haemorrhage	Complications when met are usually of minor nature, e.g. wound infection
Suitable for mass sterilization camps	Unsuitable for mass sterilization camps

procedure is mostly replaced by laparoscopic method. Currently, its place is restricted to a concurrent procedure along with any other vaginal surgery like repair for genital prolapse.

Contraindications
- Previous pelvic infection
- Previous abdominal surgery
- Suspected intra-abdominal adhesions
- Large uterus–puerperal or after second trimester MTP.

Anaesthesia
General or spinal anaesthesia.

Instruments
Instruments required for vaginal surgery.

Steps

1. After giving lithotomy position, perineum and vagina are cleaned with antiseptic solution.
2. Posterior lip of the cervix is held by volsellum forceps.
3. Posterior colpotomy is made, incising the vagina and the peritoneum.
4. Soonawalla's speculum is inserted into the vaginal incision to retract the posterior wall.
5. Right-angled retractor is introduced anteriorly through the incision to push the uterus to one side.
6. Fallopian tubes are visualized, grasped with Babcock's forceps and brought into the vagina and ligated one after the other.
7. Colpotomy wound is closed by catgut sutures.

Postoperative

a. The patient can be discharged after 6 hours.
b. Antibiotics are given prophylactically.
c. Sexual abstinence is advised for 3–4 weeks.

Advantages
- Stitchless operation from the patient's point of view
- Postopertive convalescence smooth with rapid recovery.

Disadvantages
- Tubes may not be accessible in some cases, requiring abdominal operation to complete the procedure.
- Risk of injury to rectum
- Postoperative pelvic infection is more common.
- High failure rate.

HYSTEROSCOPIC STERILIZATION

The fallopian tubes can be occluded transvaginally by:
a. Cauterization of tubal ostei
b. Introduction of ceramic or polyethylene plugs
c. Chemicals
   These methods are still in experimental stage.

CHEMICAL STERILIZATION

The chemicals used for occluding the fallopian tubes are instilled in the uterine cavity via hysteroscope under direct vision or blindly through a catheter. They may act in two ways:

- *Sclerosing agents:* Destroying the inner lining of the tube with subsequent fibrosis
- *Tissue adhesive:* Plug formation in the cornual ends of the tubes due to solidification

Quinacrine–sclerosing agent, silastic–silicon polymer and MCA–Methyl 1, 2-cyanoacrilate have been tried.

These methods have high failure rate and require multiple instillations.

Techniques of Tubal Obliteration

1. Tubal ligation
   - Simple ligation
   - Ligation and crushing–Madlener's method
   - Ligation, division and burial–Irving's method
   - Ligation and resection:
     - Pomeroy's method
     - Fimbriectomy
     - Total salpingectomy
   - Ligation, resection and burial–Uchida's method.
2. Application of clips or bands
3. Fulguration: Fulguration by monopolar cautery carries a risk of burns to intraperitoneal structures. Use of bipolar cautery is relatively safe.

Some Common Techniques

1. *Pomeroy's method:* Midportion of the tube is picked up with Babcock's forceps, the base of the loop is ligated with catgut 1/0 and the loop is cut off (Fig. 28.1).

   Advantages
   - Simple procedure
   - Less time-consuming

- As catgut gets absorbed, the severed ends of the tubes get pulled apart, thus chances of recanalization become rare, giving it a high rate of success.
- Low morbidity
- Easy reversal

Disadvantage

Failure rate is higher if performed during caesarean section.

2. *Madlener's method:* A loop of the middle portion of the tube is picked up, its base is crushed and ligated with nonabsorbable suture material.

   Disadvantage: High failure rate due to reanastomosis and regeneration of tissue at the site of crushing.

3. *Uchida method:* Epinephrine-saline solution (1:1000) is injected in the ampullary region beneath the serosa to separate it from the muscular portion of the tube. The serosa is incised, about 5 cm segment of the tube is excised between two clamps and the stumps are ligated. The medial stump is burried into the serosa while the lateral stump is left projecting into the peritoneal cavity.

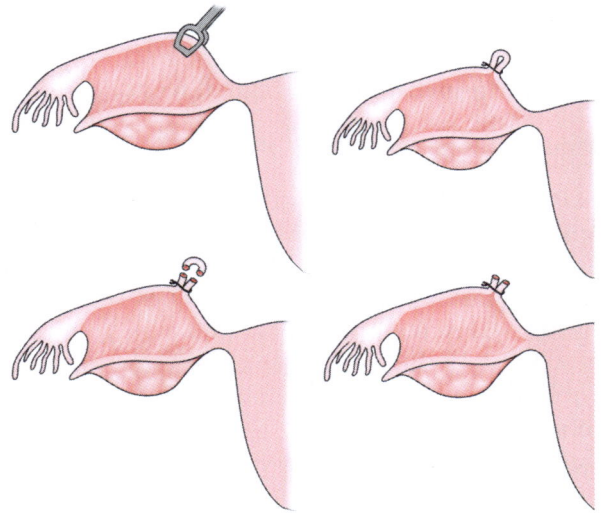

Fig. 28.1: Pomeroy's method

Disadvantage: Complicated and time consuming

Advantage: Highly effective

4. *Irving's method:* The tubes are divided near the cornual ends between two absorbable (catgut) ligatures. The proximal stump is buried in a tunnel made in the uterine musculature and the tunnel is closed over the stump. The lateral end is buried in the mesosalpinx.

Advantage: Almost 100% effective method

Disadvantages
- Technically difficult
- Time consuming
- More bleeding
- Reversal procedure difficult

5. *Kroener's method (fimbriectomy):* Distal one-third of the tubes with fimbrial ends are removed after putting a double silk ligature.

Advantages
- Success rate is almost 100%
- Easily performed through vaginal route

Disadvantage: Reversal almost impossible.

6. *Cornual resection:* A catgut ligature is placed near the uterotubal junction and the tube is dissected free from the mesosalpinx about 1 cm medial to it. A wedge of surrounding uterine myometrium is excised. The divided end of the tube is burried in the broad ligament.

Disadvantages
- Profuse bleeding
- Unsuitable for puerperal or post-abortal case
- Irreversible
- Requires laparotomy

7. *Total salpingectomy:* Both the tubes are excised at their cornual ends and the proximal uterine ends are ligated. This method usually is not performed for sterilization.

Disadvantages
- Extensive procedure
- Laparotomy required
- More bleeding
- Irreversible

VASECTOMY

Counseling

Careful and accurate counseling is essential before any man is submitted to vasectomy. The counseling should take place in a free atmosphere in a language that the man fully understands. It should be in the presence of his wife or any other person if he wishes so. Person's wife should be in reproductive age, i.e. 15–45 years of age. Following information should be delivered:

1. Description of the various temporary and permanent methods of family planning and the merits and demerits of all.
2. An explanation of the permanence of vasectomy; with clear picture of the scope and success rate of the vasovasostomy.
3. Necessity to continue some other method of contraception up to 3 months even after vasectomy; until the semen becomes azoospermic.
4. Contraindications to vasectomy and possible side effects and failure rate of vasectomy.
5. Assurance of unprejudiced family planning advice even if he withdraws his consent for vasectomy.

Contraindications

There is no absolute contraindication for vasectomy.

1. Local skin infections such as scabies or genital tract infections if present, should be treated before surgery.
2. Local pathology, making operation difficult; *viz.* varicocoele, large hydrocoele, inguinal hernia, filariasis, scar tissue of previous surgery, etc. should be looked for. Such cases

should be operated by a specialist surgeon in a well equipped hospital.

3. STDs, if present should be treated.

4. Cases of diabetes mellitus should be deferred till it is brought under control.

5. Acute febrile illness, jaundice, severe anaemia, severe hypertension, thyrotoxicosis and other chronic systemic diseases.

6. Disorders of blood coagulation.

7. Recent attack of coronary heart disease.

8. Marital, psychological or sexual instability.

Misconceptions Regarding Vasectomy

Acceptance of vasectomy is much lower compared to that of tubectomy, eventhough it is a far simpler and safer method.

- In many male dominated cultures, contraception is thought to be a woman's responsibility.
- Usually, in most of the families, man is the principle earning member; hence it is felt that he should not be exposed to any health risks or inconveniences.
- Fear of sexual problems after vasectomy is common. Many men confuse vasectomy with castration and believe that the operation will result into impotence and loss of sexual desire.
- Some believe that there is a failure to ejaculate after vasectomy.
- There is a fear that after vasectomy, men lose their physical vigour and capacity to do heavy work.

Preoperative Care

- Shaving of the parts and cleaning with antiseptic lotion. Iodine should be avoided since it causes excoriation of the scrotal skin; however povidon iodine is safe and effective.
- Proper consent in the prescribed forms. This has to be an informed consent, stating the chance of failure of the procedure resulting in unwanted, unexpected pregnancy, which if happens, can be terminated legally.

Anaesthesia

Local anaesthesia–Lignocaine 1% without adrenaline (maximum 20 ml).

Instruments

- Sponge holding forceps
- Artery forceps (mosquito)
- Allis forceps
- BP handle no. 4 with blade no. 22
- Suturing material
- Needle holding forceps

Steps of Operation

A. Conventional Vasectomy

1. Patient is made to lie in dorsal position.
2. Parts are painted and draped.
3. The vas is located and anchored:
   - The vas lies within the spermatic cord.
   - It has got a diameter of about 2.5 mm.
   - It extends from testis to the external ring in the ligament just above the pubic bone.
4. The cord is separated from the rest of the spermatic cord by gently pulling the testis downwards to draw the cord taught.
5. Vas is felt at the back of the scrotum with the thumb and fingers of one hand. The vas is a thick tube that can be rolled between the fingers. If the vas cannot be felt, then incision should not be made.
6. About 5 ml of Inj. lignocaine 1% is injected at the site of the incision under the scrotal skin and then into the sheath of the vas.
7. Two incisions of up to 2 cms are made on the scrotum on each side at the site where the vas is held taut. Alternatively, a single midline incision can be taken.
8. The vas is denuded.
9. About 1 cm portion of the vas is picked up in Allis forceps and two mosquito forceps are applied to it. The portion of

the vas between the mosquito forceps is cut and both the ends are ligated by non-absorbable sututres (2/0 silk). The knots should not be tied too tight, lest they may cut through, allowing leakage of sperms into the surrounding tissue, causing a granuloma.

10. Similar procedure is repeated on the other side.
11. Removed portion of the vas is confirmed by passing a needle through its lumen.
12. Hemostasis is ensured before closing the incision.
13. Skin is sutured by thread (Fig. 29.1 for the site of vasectomy).

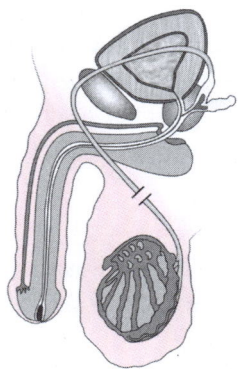

Fig. 29.1: Male reproductive system: site of vasectomy

B. *No-Scalpel Vasectomy (NSV)*

This is a method of vasectomy introduced in China.

Instruments

- Vas fixation extracutaneous ringed forceps
- Vas dissection forceps

Step

A rubber band is tied around the penis and is fixed by a clip to the patient's gown or shirt. This makes the median raphe of the scrotum taught.

Anaesthesia

- Injection lignocaine (1%) 10 ml is used for local anaesthesia.
- *Three finger technique*

- Thumb is kept at the juncture of upper and middle-thirds of median raphe.
- Middle finger is placed under the scrotum.
- Vas is palpated and swept towards the median raphe.
- The vas is held in position by thumb, middle finger and the index finger.

- Upward pressure is given by middle finger while downwards pressure is given by index finger. This creates a bend in the vas.
- A wheal is created in the skin by lignocaine. Through the wheal, the injection needle of 1.5 inches is pierced in the external spermatic fascia and the needle is proceeded parallel to the vas towards the direction of inguinal canal.
- 2.5 ml of lignocaine is injected to create the vasal block.
- The hands are changed to anaesthetize the other vas.

Vasectomy

- With the *Three Finger Technique* vas on one side is fixed and ringed forceps is applied extracutaneously to grasp the vas perpendicular to the scrotum. The handles of forceps are lowered to elevate the vas.
- A puncture is made over the vas by the median blade of dissecting forceps and then the blade is pushed into the lumen of the vas.
- The blade is withdrawn and then its whole tip is pushed inside in closed fashion.
- The forceps are opened crosswise to widen the opening.
- The sheath is also opened in the same way.
- Wall of the vas is pierced by the lateral blade of the forceps.
- The vas is brought out by rotating the forceps after removing the ringed forceps.
- A portion of the vas is removed and the ends are tied the same way as in the conventional vasectomy technique.
- The vas is pushed in.
- The same procedure is carried out on the opposite side.

- After completion of vasectomy, the puncture site is pinched to achieve the haemostasis.
- Skin suturing is not required.

Advantages
- Less invasive and less time consuming
- Faster recovery
- Less painful
- Less bleeding and hence, less chances of haematoma formation
- Less chances of infection
- Lesser postoperative complications
- Higher acceptability.

Postoperative Care

1. Rest for a couple of hours in the clinic
2. Rest for a day at home
3. Avoid hard work or strenuous exercise for two to three days after surgery
4. Avoid driving vehicles like bicycle, sitting astride; for 8 days
5. Wear scrotal support for a week
6. Use of mild analgesics, if required
7. Abstinence period depends upon personal discomfort. As soon as the man feels comfortable, he can have sexual intercourse.

Contraception after Vasectomy

Vasectomy, unlike tubectomy, does not result in immediate infertility. Sperms stored in the male reproductive tract on the distal to the site of vasectomy must be expelled out before the couple goes for unprotected sexual intercourse. It takes about 6 to 12 weeks or 15 to 20 ejaculations for all those sperms to get expelled out completely. It is therefore, advisable to instruct the vasectomised man to use some other method of contraception like condom until the semen analysis confirms the absence of sperms.

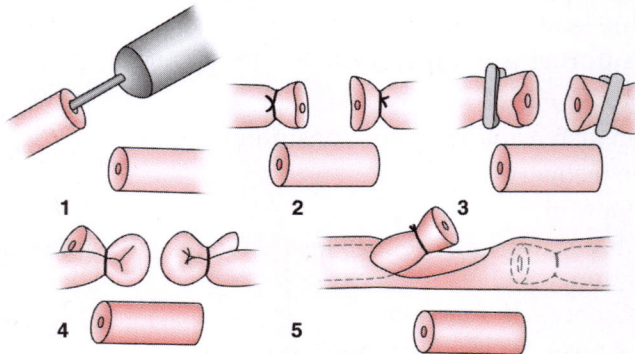

Fig. 29.2: Various techniques of sealing vas. 1. Mucousal electro-coagulation; 2. Removal of segment and simple ligation; 3. Removal of segment and tantalum clips application; 4. Removal of segment and turning both ends on themselves; 5. Removal of segment, ligation and closing fascia over one end

Effectiveness

Vasectomy failures are usually due to:
- Unprotected coitus before all the sperms distal to the site of vasectomy are ejaculated
- Spontaneous recanalization of the vas
- Division and occlusion of the wrong structure during vasectomy
- Rarely, congenital duplication of the vas that had gone unnoticed during vasectomy.

Techniques for Preventing Reunion of Vas

a. Removal of the segment and simple ligation (Fig. 29.2)
b. Doubling back of the vas and suturing on to itself
c. Turning the ends from each other
d. Pulling the sheath of the vas over one end to create a barrier of fascial tissue.

Complications and Side Effects

1. *Short-term:* Immediate complications of vasectomy are usually minor and most of them subside within a week or two.

a. Swelling

b. *Bruising:* It is usually caused by seepage of blood under the skin where the anaesthetic needle punctures small blood vessels.

c. *Pain:* Many patients experience tenderness and dragging sensation in the scrotum for up to a week after vasectomy. Surgical manipulation of scrotal tissue and subsequent swelling cause this discomfort. Scrotal support and analgesics relieve these discomforts. Severe pain indicates infection or haematoma formation.

d. *Haematoma:* When blood vessels in the subcutaneous layer of the scrotum are injured and bleed into the scrotal sac, haematoma is formed. The scrotal tissue being lax, continues to expand, resulting in more bleeding; forming a large haematoma. If haematoma is not treated, pain and infection can result.

Prevention of Haematoma

- Proper haemostasis should be achieved during surgery.
- Patient must not strain the scrotal sac for several days after surgery.
- Patient should rest after the procedure and avoid strenuous work for two days.
- Patient should use scrotal support for at least six weeks after the procedure.
- Small haematomata usually require no active treatment and get completely absorbed with complete bed rest. Larger haematomata may require drainage.

e. *Infection:* Skin infection at the site of the scrotal incision or skin sutures is most common, particularly when non-absorbable sutures are used. Deep infections of vas and epididymis are vary rare, but can occur up to six months later and may require prolonged antibiotic treatment.
Treatment of infection depends upon its severity. Superficial infections at the wound site usually heal without treatment. If pus forms around the incision, it should be allowed to drain. In such cases, skin sutures may have to

be removed and antibiotic should be started. In rare instances an abscess may require opening and drainage.

f. *Allergic reaction:* Rarely, the patient may show an allergic response to local anaesthetic and may even land into an anaphylactic shock. It is advisable to test the local anaesthetic for allergy, and also to keep medicines like corticosteroids ready.

g. *Sperm granuloma:* It is a non-bacterial abscess consisting largely of sperms, epithelial cells and lymphocytes. It is an inflammatory response to sperms leaking into surrounding tissue and can occur either at the site of vasectomy or in the epididymis. Usually, the granulomata are small and nonsignificant, however, very occasionally following problems may arise:

- Channels may develop through the granuloma, forming a new passageway for sperms, restoring fertility.
- Rarely, sperm granuloma might give rise to pain.
- Epididymal granuloma may prevent successful vasectomy reversal.
- Up to 10% of the men with sperm granuloma get some symptoms. The most common symptom is tender nodule at the cut end of the vas or in the epididymis. Some develop discomfort at the site of granuloma particularly during sexual excitement or ejaculation. In most cases, this discomfort subsides spontaneously. Conservative treatment with mild analgesics or anti-inflammatory medication and bed rest is often enough. In rare cases, sperm granulomata may require surgical evacuation and if necessary, resealing of the testicular end of the vas.

2. *Long-term risks:* Vasectomy carries little if any long-term risk to human physical or mental health. However, the following points are being studied in this respect (Table 29.1)

a. Development of atherosclerosis

b. Affection of the immune system due to constant antibody response to sperms, increasing the risk of autoimmune diseases

Table 29.1: Comparison of vasectomy and female sterilization

Vasectomy	*Female sterilization*
Effectiveness	
• Effective 6–10 wks after surgery	• Effective immediately after surgery
• Failure rate up to 1%	• Failure rate 0.1% to 0.4%
Complications	
• More safe	• Comparatively higher risk of major complications and internal injuries
• No risk of major complications and internal injury	• Slightly higher risk of serious infections
• Possibility of serious infection is remote	• Some anaesthetic deaths are known
• No anaesthesia related complications except occasional allergic reaction to local anaesthetic	
Acceptability	
• Less expensive	• More expensive
• Minute scar	• Scar relatively larger, except in laparoscopic sterilization
• Abdomen not opened	• Peritoneal cavity is opened
• Reversal more successful	• Poor potential for reversal
Personal	
• Easier procedure	• Comparatively less easy
• Less time required	• Relatively more time required
• Local anaesthesia	• Local or general anaesthesia
Backup facility	
• No additional facilities required	• To manage complications, backup facilities required
Long-term risks	
• No definite long-term risks	• Slightly higher risk of ectopic pregnancy

c. Prostatic malignancy

However, so far, none of these effects have been convincingly demonstrated in man.

Drugs

30. Drugs in Obstetrics and Gynaecology

Drugs in Obstetrics and Gynaecology

NUTRITIONAL ANAEMIA COMPLICATING PREGNANCY

Usually anaemias complicating pregnancy are due to nutritional deficiency (iron, folic acid, B_{12} deficiency).

ORAL IRON

Prophylaxis of Iron Deficiency Anaemia

Oral tablets containing 100 mg elemental iron and 0.5 mg folic acid are recommended under national RCH programme, 1 tablet daily for minimum 100 days.

Usually recommended to take throughout pregnancy from second trimester and continued during lactation.

Correction of Anaemia

1 tab 2–3 times daily

Side Effects

Symptoms of intolerance–abdominal cramps, constipation, diarrhoea.

Effects of Oral Iron

- Subjective well-being: 3–4 days
- Increase in reticulocyte count: 5–7 days
- Rise in haemoglobin: 2–3 weeks
- Rate of Hb rise: 1 gm% every week

If no response after 4–6 weeks–confirm about intake of medicine–ask for colour of stools–stools turn black.

Causes of Non-response
- Poor patient compliance.
- GIT problems leading to malabsorption.
- Other causes of anaemia.
- Refractory anaemia due to chronic infections.

PARENTERAL IRON
Iron Sucrose
2.5 ml/5 ml ampoule containing 50 mg/100 mg of elemental iron as iron sucrose. Each dose may be administered as slow IV injection. 100 mg injected IV over 2–5 minutes or IV infusion 5 ml iron sucrose diluted in 100 ml of normal saline, and infused IV at a rate of 100 mg of iron over a period of at least 15 minutes. Each dose of 100 mg IV may be repeated up to 3 times per week.

Use
Iron deficiency anaemia with following conditions:
- Noncompliant patient
- Intolerance to oral iron
- GIT problems hindering iron absorption.

Advantages
- Assured administration
- Builds up iron stores fast.
- Generally safe

Side Effects
Occasionally: hypotension, chest pain, cramps, musculoskeletal pain, GIT upset may occur.

IRON DEXTRAN (IMFERON)
Available as 50 mg/ml injection

Disadvantages
- Possibility of anaphylaxis

- Painful injection
- Staining of the skin

Rate of Hb rise after parenteral iron therapy is not significantly different as compared to that of oral iron.

Dose and Administration

- IM or IV–intermittent or total dose infusion
- Absorbed through lymphatics
- Total iron required =

  $(0.3 \times \text{wt in lb} \times \text{Hb deficit\%}) + 500 \text{ mg}$

  Addition of 500 mg for replenishing the stores.
- *Sensitivity test:* Test dose of 0.5 ml is injected deep IM, wait for 24 hours.
- 100 mg deep IM (in buttocks) on alternate days by Z technique to avoid staining of the skin.

IRON SORBITOL CITRIC ACID COMPLEX (JECTOFER)
Dose and Administration

Available as 75 mg/1.5 cc in an ampoule for intramuscular use only.

Precautions

- Oral iron must be discontinued at least 48 hours before starting.
- Avoided in patients with impaired renal function
- Since 30% of the injected drug is excreted in urine, the required dose is more.

Toxicity

- Nausea
- Vomiting
- Diarrhoea
- Pain in joints
- Myalgia

FOLIC ACID
Indications

- Along with oral iron for prophylaxis of nutritional anaemia during pregnancy (0.4 mg daily)
- Megaloblastic anaemia
- Periconceptional folic acid therapy 400 mcg daily protective for first occurrence of open neural tube defects (NTD) like anencephaly. Recurrence markedly reduced with 4 mg daily.

PREECLAMPSIA–ECLAMPSIA

ANTIHYPERTENSIVE DRUGS
Indication

Severe diastolic hypertension >110 mm of Hg

Aim

To prevent maternal complications of severe diastolic hypertension such as cerebral haemorrhage. Most of the drugs reduce the placental perfusion with resultant lowering of birth weight and as such do not have any beneficial effect on foetus.

Drugs Suggested

- Alpha Methyl Dopa
- Nifedipine
- Hydrallazine
- Atenelol
- Labetelol

Since sudden drop in BP can reduce placental perfusion with detrimental effects on foetus, diastolic pressure should be maintained around 90–100 mm of Hg.

ALPHA METHYL DOPA
Mode of Action

- Effectively inhibits the decarboxylation of both dopa and 5- HT

- Decreases the concentration of 5-HT, dopamine and norepinephrine in CNS

  Onset of action after 1–2 hours; however, erratic onset of action is observed.

  Maximum reduction in BP is seen at 4–6 hours.

Dose and Administration

250 mg tablet: One tablet thrice a day.

The dose can be increased up to 500 mg 6 hourly.

Advantage

Does not affect circulation to vital organs.

Side Effects

- *Maternal:* Sedation, vertigo, depression, extrapyramidal symptoms
- *Foetal:* Reduced birth weight

NIFEDIPINE

Mode of Action

- Calcium channel blocker.
- Direct action on blood vessels–relaxes the arterial smooth muscles.

Dose and Administration

Oral: 10–20 mg every 6–8 hours

Onset of action 20 minutes and peak action reached in 1 hour.

Side Effects

- Headache
- Dizziness

Advantages

- Does not affect the perfusion of vital organs.
- Does not affect cardiac preload

NIMODIPINE

Calcium channel blocker having greater action on the cerebral vessels. Hence it is used in severe PIH and eclampsia.

Dose and Administration

30 mg 6–8 hourly orally

ATENELOL

Mode of Action

β-blocker

Dose and Administration

25–50 mg twice a day orally

LABETELOL

Mode of Action

α and β-blocker
Prefered drug as it does not affect the cerebral autoregulation

Dose and Administration

50 mg twice a day orally

LABETELOL IV (AVOID IN ASTHMA)

10 mg initial, 20 mg if BP still high after 10 min, 20 and 40 mg if required every 10 min (max total dose 220 mg).

Anti-hypertensive Drugs *not* Recommended during Pregnancy	
1. Reserpine	Maternal depression, foetal bradycardia, neonatal hypothermia
2. Diuretics	Aggravate haemoconcentration, reduced birth weight
3. Propranolol	IUGR, neonatal hypoglycemia, apnoea
4. ACE inhibitors	Risk of neonatal renal failure
5. Angiotensin receptor blocking agents	

DIURETICS

Indications

1. CCF due to:
   - Severe anaemia
   - Rheumatic valvular heart disease
2. Pulmonary oedema
3. Suspected fluid overload
4. Oliguria suggestive of impending renal failure in PET, eclampsia, placental abruption, etc. for differentiation of prerenal causes from renal causes after fluid challenge
5. Before blood transfusion in cases of severe anaemia.

Drug of Choice

Frusemide

20–40 mg IV. Can be repeated if necessary.

In preeclampsia, diuretics are indicated only when there is pulmonary oedema or impending renal failure.

Thiazide diuretics given near the time of delivery can cause neonatal thrombocytopenia.

ANTICONVULSANT DRUGS IN ECLAMPSIA

Magnesium sulfate is the safe and effective drug for controlling convulsions in eclampsia.

Other drugs used in past: Diazepam, phenytoin sodium and lytic cocktail regime consisting of Pethidine + Largactyl + Phenergan.

MAGNESIUM SULFATE

Mode of Action

- Neuromuscular conduction is slowed, decreased neuronal burst firing
- Calcium entry is blocked
- Blocks neuromuscular transmission by decreasing acetyl choline release and reducing sensitivity of end plate to acetyl choline.

Dose and Administration

Prichard Regime

- *Initial loading dose:* 20 ml of 20% (4 gm) MgSO$_4$ to be given intravenously over a period of 3 minutes.
- *This is immediately followed by:* 20 ml of 50% (10 gm) MgSO$_4$ intramuscularly in two divided doses–one on each buttock to be given one after the other.
- *Maintenance dose:* 10 ml of 50% (5 gm) every four hours on alternate buttocks.

Precaution

To avoid adverse effects due to hypermagnesia, ensure the following before every subsequent dose

- Knee jerk must be present.
- Urine output should be >= 100 ml in previous 4 hours
- Respiratory rate should be about 16/minute. If there are signs of respiratory depression, the next dose is withheld and respiratory depression is treated by 10 ml intravenous injection of 10% calcium gluconate.

IV Regime

A loading dose of 4 g by infusion pump over 5–10 minutes, followed by a further infusion of 1 g/hour maintained for 24 hours after the last seizure.

Recurrent seizures treated with either a further bolus of 2 g magnesium sulphate or an increase in the infusion rate to 1.5 g or 2.0 g/hour.

Low Dose Regimes

To minimize toxicity in women with low BMI various low dose regimes have been tried and found to be safe and effective, e.g. 10 gm loading followed by 2.5 gm IM 4 hourly, for 24 hours. Slightly higher recurrences of fits observed.

The anticonvulsant treatment is to be continued until 24 hours after the last convulsion/delivery.

Advantages
>   i. Patient remains conscious and alert
>   ii. Effective control of convulsions
> iii. No adverse effect on foetus.

Uses

- Control of convulsions in eclampsia
- Prevention of convulsions in severe pre-eclampsia.

PHENYTOIN SODIUM

Dose and Administration

10 mg/kg body weight
> Diluted in normal saline and administered IV slowly

Side effects: Arrhythmias and hypotension; hence respiratory and cardiac monitoring essential.

Advantage: No maternal or foetal CNS depression.

Disadvantage: Control of convulsions inferior to $MgSO_4$.

DIAZEPAM

Mode of Action

- Depressant action on brainstem reticular formation
- Skeletal muscle relaxant
- Sedative, hypnotic and anticonvulsant action

Because of adverse effects on mother and baby and inferior control of fits in comparison to MgSO4 the diazepam regime is not recommended for use in eclampsia. It can be given before referral or for arresting fits if the fits recur after $MgSO_4$ injection.

Dose and Administration

5–10 mg is given IV over 2–4 minutes. The anticonvulsant action lasts for 15–20 minutes.

Adverse Effects

1. *Maternal:*
>   i. Respiratory depression

  ii. Bradycardia, hypotension, cardiovascular collapse
 iii. Paradoxical hyperexcitability.
2. *Foetal and neonatal:* The neonate cannot metabolize the drug.
   i. Decreased foetal heart variability
  ii. Neonatal depression leading to apnoeic spells and may require laryngeal intubation. This may necessitate admission to neonatal intensive care units
 iii. Hypotonia
  iv. Neonatal hypotension
   v. Impaired neonatal thermoregulation
  vi. Poor sucking reflex
 vii. Neonatal withdrawal syndrome
viii. Hyperbilirubinaemia
  ix. Terratogenic effect–oral clefts.

LYTIC COCKTAIL

Dr. Krishna Menon introduced this regime for treatment of eclampsia.

Drug Combination

Pethidine + Chlorpromazine + Promethazine

Limitations

- Control of convulsions less effective–recurrence in 15%
- Maternal CNS depression
- Foetal depression–high PNM (30%)
  This regime is not recommended.

ASPIRIN

- Low dose aspirin (60–80 mg daily) is used in recurrent foetal wastages due to antiphospholipid syndrome ; Aspirin 75 mg daily is used in combination with Heparin or Prednisone.
- Low dose aspirin is effective in prevention of pregnancy induced hypertension for women at highest risk from previous severe preeclampsia, diabetes, chronic hypertension, renal or autoimmune disease.

Problems: Oligohydramnios, premature closure of fetal ductus arteriosus and pulmonary oedema.

Mode of Action

- Cyclooxygenase inhibitor (antiprostaglandin effect)
- Reduces production of thromboxane A_2 by platelets.

Dose and Administration

75–100 mg daily orally. To be discontinued few weeks prior to the expected date of delivery.

OXYTOCIC DRUGS

OXYTOCIN

Uses

Therapeutic

- Induction of labour
- Augmentation of labour in slow progress of labour due to hypotonic uterine action
- Prevention of atonic PPH
- Control of atonic PPH
- Augmentation of second trimester abortion.

Diagnostic

- Contraction stress test
- Oxytocin sensitivity test

Mode of Administration

IV infusion

For Induction/Augmentation of Labour

Dose: 1 to 5 mIU/min

2 to 5 IU added to 500 ml of N. saline/Ringer's lactate. Initially 8 drops per min (2 to 5 mIU/min) is infused. Infusion rate is increased by 8 drops per min. every 30 mins until optimum response seen.

Low concentration (0.5 to 1.5 mU/min) and high concentration infusions (5 mU/min) are used. With proper monitoring high dose infusions are safe.

Escalating technique: Dose is increased every 30 min. until optimum response is observed. (Three contractions in 10 minutes, each lasting for 45 seconds.)

Action: Oxytocin enhances the normal pattern of uterine contractions with intermittent relaxation.

Contraindications

- CPD
- Malpresentations
- Foetal distress
- Scar on the uterus

Monitoring

Every 15 minutes, following parameters are monitored:
- Drip rate
- Uterine contractions–frequency and intensity
- FHR
- Maternal pulse
- Progress of labour is checked periodically.

Complications

- Hypertonic uterine contractions (contraction lasting >90 seconds), uterus failing to relax between the contractions, Tachysystole: 6 or more uterine contractions/10 minutes, hyperstimulation : Excessive uterine activity associated with FHR abnormalities
- Foetal bradycardia (distress)
- Uterine rupture–if drip is not supervised vigilantly
- Water intoxication if too much of electrolyte free infusion is administered (with dose above 40–50 mU/min)
- Neonatal hyperbilirubinaemia.

Treatment of Hyperstimulation

- Discontinue the drip
- Maternal repositioning

- O$_2$ therapy
- IV tocolysis if required.

Caution

i. Maximum concentration should not exceed 40 mIU/min.
ii. Maximum drip rate should not exceed 60 drops/min lest the risk of water intoxication.
iii. Cautious use in multiparous women as the uterus tends to rupture easily.

Six hours of strong stimulated uterine activity unable to bring progress of labour → discontinue the drip and review the case.

For induction and augmentation of labour, the drug should **never** be given intramuscularly.

For PPH

Intramuscular Oxytocin 5–10 IU at the delivery of anterior shoulder/soon after birth of newborn is useful in prevention of atonic PPH in active management of third stage of labor.

Oxytocin 10–20 IU in 500 ml of normal saline can be given at the rate of 40 drops/min for prevention or control of atonic PPH.

METHYL ERGOMETRINE

Uses

- Prevention of atonic PPH
- Control of atonic PPH

Dose and Administration

0.2 mg administered IV at the delivery of anterior shoulder helps in prevention of PPH.

Action

Intramuscular: After 3–7 minutes

After administration of methyl ergotamine, uterus contracts tonically; also the cervix tends to close. Action lasts longer.

Contraindications

1. *Hypertension:* IV bolus dose of ergot preparation can lead to acute hypertension.
2. *Cardiac disease:* Too short third stage will diverge about 500 ml of blood from uteroplacental bed to systemic circulation; thus precipitating cardiac failure.
3. *Suspected multiple pregnancy:* Ergot preparation should be with-held until the last baby is delivered; lest risk of severe asphyxia of unborn fetus.
4. *Rh incompatibility:* To minimize the amount of foetomaternal haemorrhage thus to minimize the chances of sensitization.

PROSTAGLANDINS

CARBOPROST TROMETHAMINE (15 METHYL PGF$_2$-α)
Dose and Administration

- Prevention of PPH–125 μg IM at the delivery of anterior shoulder
- For control of PPH–250 μg IM or intramyometrial; can be repeated every 15 minutes.

Other Uses

- Induction of second trimester abortion
- Preoperative cervical dilatation before suction evacuation for first trimester MTP.

Side Effects

- Nausea and vomiting
- Diarrhoea
- Chills
- Pyrexia

Contraindications

Bronchial asthma, hypertension, cardiac disease, scar on uterus, renal disease.

DINOPROSTONE

PGE_2 oral tablets 0.5 mg.

Use

For induction of labour.

Side Effects

Nausea and vomiting, diarrhoea, fever.

Advantages

Facilitates cervical ripening, avoids IV drip.

Disadvantage

No precision of control on administration.

DINOPROSTONE GEL

Available as 0.5 mg in a prefilled syringe.

Use

- Preinduction cervical ripening in cases with unripe cervix, i.e. Bishop score <= 5

Dose and Administration

0.5 mg endocervical instillation. Bishop score is increased after 12–24 hours of instillation. Around 30%–40% patients go in labour with Cerviprime only. The rest can have successful induction with oxytocin drip.

Caution

- Avoid instillation of the drug beyond internal os
- Monitor uterine contractions and FHR for 1 hour.

Risk

Hyperstimulation: Excessive uterine activity with foetal brady-cardia.

MISOPROSTOL (PGE$_1$ TABLETS)

- Available as 25, 50, 100 and 200 mcg tablets for oral use.
- Can be administered by vaginal or rectal route
- Cheap, stable at room temperature

Uses

- *Induction of labor:* 25 to 50 mcg 3 to 6 hourly by vaginal route, maximum 4 doses.

  Side effects tachysystole, fetal distress, uterine rupture.

  In women with previous cesarean delivery or major uterine surgery, the use of misoprostol should be avoided as there is higher risk of uterine rupture.
- Medical termination of pregnancy in first trimester as part of sequential regime with Mifepristone.
- Active management of third stage of labor (prevention of atonic PPH): 600 mcg oral soon after birth of baby (less effective than oxytocin or methergine.

  The comparison of oxytocic agents is shown in Tables 30.1 and 30.2.

TOCOLYTIC DRUGS

- β-agonist: Isoxsuprine, Ritodrine, Terbutaline, Salbutamol
- MgSO$_4$

Table 30.1: Oxytocin and ergot alkaloids	
Oxytocin	*Ergot preparations*
• Effects physiological uterine contractions followed by relaxation.	• Effect tonic contractions of the uterus.
• Maintains normal polarity. Effects cervical dilatation.	• Cervix tends to close
• Hence it can be safely used for induction and augmentation of labour	• Hence it cannot be used before delivery.
• Can be used for controlling atonic PPH	• Highly effective for preventing and controlling atonic PPH
• IV bolus can cause hypotension and bradycardia	• IV bolus dose can cause acute hypertension

Table 30.2: Comparison of oxytocin and prostaglandins

Oxytocin	Prostaglandins
Effective on ripe cervix	Can effect cervical ripening; hence effective on unripe cervix also
Effective on women who are near term; hence not useful for pregnancy termination in earlier weeks.	Effective at all stages of pregnancy; therefore can be used for MTP.
Administration by IV infusion	Different preparations can be administered by different routes. (oral, IM, endocervical, vaginal); hence patient comfortable
Precision of control	Once administered, cannot be withdrawn.
Safe in all cases; can be used under expert supervision on scarred uterus also.	$PGF_{2\alpha}$ Contraindicated in systemic diseases and bronchial asthma. Use avoided in scarred uterus.
No side effects	Troublesome GIT side effects on oral use. Less with vaginal and endocervical use

- Nifedipine
- Indomethacin
- Nitrous oxide donors–glyceryl trinitrate
- Oxytocin inhibitors–atociban

Indications

1. Preterm labour
2. Uterine hyperstimulation caused by oxytocics
3. External cephalic version–improved success.

Prerequisites for Use of Tocolytic Drugs

- Unexplained preterm labour
- Healthy mother
- Normal healthy foetus
- Gestational age not more than 34 weeks
- Estimated foetal weight <1500–2000 gm (depends upon the salvageability in a given set up)

- Intact membranes
- Cervical dilatation not more than 3 cm

Exclude conditions where continuation of pregnancy is not advisable, e.g. foetal death, foetal malformations incompatible with life, premature rupture of membranes, chorioamnionitis, etc.

Value

Can postpone labour but do not improve neonatal outcome significantly. There is no clear evidence that they improve outcome. However, tocolysis should be considered for gaining few days for completing a course of corticosteroids, or in utero transfer to better care facility.

Maintenance therapy not recommended for routine practice.

Inhibitory Drugs could be Potentially Harmful

All the drugs have inherent risks, however benefits for the baby should outweigh the risks. Maternal and neonatal risk profile of each drug should be carefully reviewed before prescribing

1. *Indomethacin:* Risk of premature closure of foetal ductus arteriosus leading to pulmonary hypertension in baby
2. *MgSO₄ parenteral:* Hypermagnesemia (respiratory depression, weakness, diplopia, muscular paralysis, cardiac arrest).

Choice of Drug

Nifedipine or Atosiban appear preferable as they have fewer adverse effects and seem to have comparable effectiveness.

β–SYMPATHOMIMETIC DRUGS
Mode of Action

- *β-receptor stimulant:* The drug binds to β-adrenergic receptors on the outer cell membrane of smooth muscle and activates adenylate cyclase which converts ATP to cyclic AMP

Adenylate cyclase

$\downarrow$

ATP $\rightarrow$ Cyclic AMP

Sequestration of Ca^{++} in sarcoplasmic
reticulum leads to uterine relaxation

- Direct action on myometrium; it is a smooth muscle relaxant.

Contraindications

Absolute

- High cardiac output states, e.g. thyrotoxicosis, sickle cell disease as there is risk of pulmonary oedema.
- Chronic cardiac diseases
- Should not be used with MAO inhibiting agents.

Relative

Insulin dependent diabetes mellitus.

Adverse Effects

I. Maternal

- *Vasodilatation:* Tachycardia, palpitations, restlessness, headache, anxiety and occasionally angina pectoris.
- GI disturbances like nausea, vomiting, constipation
- Hyperglycaemia
- Hypokalaemia
- Myocardial ischemia, arrhythmias, and even maternal death.
- Pulmonary oedema due to:
  - Prolonged infusion leading to myocardial necrosis
  - Effect on pulmonary capillary endothelium causing leakage into pulmonary alveoli
  - Stimulation of β-adrenergic reaction: This leads to increase in renin concentration and thus secondary fluid retention. Maternal infection increases the risk.

β-mimetic drugs + corticosteroids can precipitate acute pulmonary oedema.

II. *Neonatal*

Hypokalaemia, hypoglycaemia, hypotension, paralytic ileus, respiratory distress syndrome, periventricular–intraventricular hemorrhage.

Selective β_2 Agonists

Terbutaline

- 0.25 mg subcutaneously 6 hourly
- Can be used IV for acute intrapartum foetal distress.

Ritodrine HCl

IV infusion

- *Initial dose:* 50 µg/min, increase by 50 µg/min every 10 min until contractions cease or maternal heart rate reaches 140 beats/min
- Effective dose 50 µg–100 µg/min (max 350 µg/min)
- Continue for 12–48 hours after contractions stop
- After 12 hours: Switch over to oral therapy.

Oral Tablets (10 mg)

- One tablet 30 min before the infusion is stopped
- 1 tablet every 2 hours for 48 hours, 10–20 mg 4 to 6 hourly.

Salbutamol

- *Intravenous infusion:* 5 mg in 5% dextrose 10 µg/min increased up to maximum 50 µg/min
- *Oral:* 4 mg every 6 hours

BOTH β_1 AND β_2 AGONIST

Isoxsuprine HCl

Dose and Administration

1. *Oral:* 30–60 mg daily in 3 divided doses
2. *Intramuscular:* 10 mg followed by two doses of 10 mg at the intervals of 2 hours and 6 hours respectively as loading dose.

Later the same dose is continued 6 hourly till the uterus is relaxed. Then the patient can be switched over to oral regime.

3. *Intravenous:* 0.02% solution is prepared by adding 100 mg isoxsuprine in 500 ml of 5% dextrose saline. 0.2 to 1 mg is given over 10 minutes as loading dose which is followed by 0.1–0.3 mg/min for 12 hours.

4. During IV administration, pulse and BP is monitored for the risk of tachycardia and hypotension.

Adverse Effects

As it is both β_1 and β_2 agonist, side effects are more. Hence, selective β_2 agonist drugs like Terbutaline, Ritodrine, Salbutamol are preferred.

NIFEDIPINE
Mode of Action

Calcium channel blocker

Dose and Administration

20 mg initial 10–20 mg/4–6 hourly.

Advantages

- *Better efficacy:* Compared with ritodrine has higher delaying of delivery for >48 hrs.
- *Good safety profile:* Lower risk of RDS and neonatal jaundice, lower admission to neonatal ICU
- Fewer maternal adverse effects
- Cheap, ease of administration by oral route
- When tocolysis is indicated for women in preterm labor, calcium channel blockers are preferable to other tocolytic agents compared, mainly with betamimetics.

MAGNESIUM SULFATE
Mode of Action

- It antagonizes action of intracellular calcium and acetyl choline
- Direct depressant action on the smooth muscles.

Dose and Administration

4 gm given intravenously (20 ml of 20% solution) slowly over 3 minutes as loading dose. This is followed by 2 gm/hour until uterine contractions cease.

Caution: Vigilant supervision is necessary on respiratory rate, knee jerk and urine output.

Disadvantage

Narrow margin of safety

Toxicity: Hypermagnesia leading to respiratory arrest or cardiac arrest

$MgSO_4$ is ineffective at delaying birth or preventing preterm birth.

INDOMETHACIN
Mode of Action

Antiprostaglandin

Dose

50 mg loading dose, then 25–50 mg/6 hrs

Fetal risks: Risk of premature closure of ductus arteriorus leading to pulmonary hypertension in baby, renal and cerebral vasoconstriction. Necrotising enterocolitis. Risks more with high dose and prolonged exposure.

Indomethacin therapy for <48 hours, not >200 mg/day and restricted to <30–32 weeks' gestation reduces the fetal risks.

Fewer maternal adverse effects than the beta-agonists.

Indomethacin may be a first-line tocolytic in associated polyhydramnios.

NITROGLYCERIN
Mode of Action

Endogenous nitrous oxide (NO) is smooth muscle relaxant. Increased synthesis of NO is associated with arrest of labour. Therefore, NO donors like nitroglycerin have been tried orally and transdermally as uterine relaxant. Found to be less effective than β-sympathomimetics.

ATOCIBAN

A synthetic peptide, is a competitive antagonist of oxytocin at uterine oxytocin receptors. Has fewer maternal adverse effects than beta-agonists and is effective as other tocolytics.

Administration Schedule

Initial bolus dose of 6.75 mg over one minute, followed by an infusion of 18 mg/hour for three hours and then 6 mg/hour for up to 45 hours. Duration of treatment should not exceed 48 hours and the total dose should not exceed 330 mg of atosiban.

TOXOPLASMOSIS DURING PREGNANCY

Spiramycin is given in acute maternal infection diagnosed during pregnancy to prevent foetal infection. Spiramycin used alone, can reduce the risk of congenital infection, but not useful to treat the established fetal infection.

Pyrimethamine/sulfadiazine is added to Spiramycin after 20 weeks of pregnancy in cases seroconverting in late pregnancy and with confirmed fetal affection. To counter the possible effects of pyrimethamine on the bone marrow, folinic acid is given along with pyrimethamine. Treatment can reduce congenital symptoms by 70%.

Spiramycin (Rovamycin Forte) 3 MIU 1 tab 2–3 times daily, orally for 4 weeks repeat after 4 weeks.

Pyrimethamine 25 mg daily, **Sulfonamide 3–4 gm** daily and folinic acid.

Monitoring: Weekly estimation of platelet count, WBC, PCV.

Side effects
- Thrombocytopenia
- Leukopenia
- Anaemia
- GIT distress
- Headache

The therapy has shown to decrease but not eliminate the incidence of congenital infection.

The therapy is administered to prevent the organism from infecting the foetus and not erradicating established disease.

PREVENTION OF HEPATITIS B

Hepatitis B Immunoglobin (HBIG)

High Risk Personnel

1. Newborn of a mother who is HbsAg positive → 0.5 ml IM as soon as possible but not later than 48 hours after the birth
2. Health care provider who sustains a contaminated needle prick injury → 0.06 ml/kg of body weight IM immediately.

Active Immunization Against Hepatitis B

Preparations: Engerix B, Enivac HB

Indications

- Newborn and infants: 0.5 ml IM
  At birth, 1 month and 6 months
- Health care providers and sexual consorts of HbsAg positive individuals
  3 doses 1 ml IM each at 0, 1 and 6 months.

CORTICOSTEROIDS

Indications

Obstetrics

1. Anaphylactic shock
   - Drug induced, e.g. Penicillin, Imferon
   - Blood transfusion reaction
2. Enhance lung maturity of foetus in preterm labour to reduce the chances of respiratory distress syndrome leading to neonatal death.
   - Betamethazone 12 mg IM, repeated 12 hours later
   - Effective after 24 hours of administration.
   - Effect lasts for about 7 days. Dose should not be repeated.
   - Most beneficial between 28–32 weeks of gestation

3. Recurrent abortions due to autoimmune aetiology
4. Antiphospholipid syndrome:
   - Tab Prednisolone 20–40 mg daily in combination with low dose aspirin (<=100 mg)
5. Systemic lupus erythematosus

Gynaecology

1. Substitution therapy for congenital adrenal hyperplasia.
2. Adjuvant therapy with ovulation inducing agents–if clomiphene citrate fails in inducing the ovulation and the cause appears to be hyperandrogenism of adrenal origin as suggested by elevated DHEAS levels.
3. Topical use in pruritus vulvae due to vulval dystrophy.
4. Prevent development of adhesions during tubal microsurgery – hydrocortisone and heparin is added to irrigating fluid.
5. Evaluation of hirsuitism–Dexamethazone suppression test.
6. Hydrotubation following tubal reconstructive surgery.

ANTICOAGULANT DRUGS

Heparin

Available as 1000 and 5000 IU injections.

Low molecular weight heparin is superior and is used for prophylactic purposes every 12 hours.

Does not cross placental barrier.

Indications

Obstetrics

1. Prophylaxis of deep vein thrombosis (DVT) in women with history of DVT or pulmonary embolism during previous pregnancies: Subcut 5000 IU 8–12 hourly
2. Deep vein thrombosis
3. Pelvic thrombophlebitis
4. Postoperative pulmonary embolism
   - Loading dose 5000–10000 IU given IV
   - Followed by infusion of 1000–2000 IU/hour

5. *Pregnancy following cardiac surgery with prosthetic heart valves:* Continued throughout pregnancy, stopped before delivery, restarted next day following delivery.
6. Recurrent pregnancy wastage due to antiphospholipid syndrome
   - Low dose aspirin: Safe and effective
   - Aspirin + Heparin 10000 IU subcut 12 hourly
   - Heparin alone also has been used
7. To block process of DIC in cases of fetal death
   Dose adjusted by activated PTT done 6 hours after injection which should be 1.5 to 2.5 times of baseline value. Use of clotting time can result in underdosage leading to thrombus extension.

Gynaecology

1. *Tubal reconstructive microsurgery:* Irrigating fluid used during surgery contains 5000 units of heparin and hydrocortisone to minimise adhesions formation.

Contraindications

Bleeding tendencies.

Side effects
- Leucopenia
- Thrombocytopenia
- Haemorrhage (overdose)
- Osteoporosis with prolonged therapy.

Antidote

Protamine sulfate 1–1.5 mg/1 mg of heparin.

PREVENTION OF RH ISOIMMUNIZATION

Anti-D Immunoglobulin

When administered at the time of delivery, it prevents 99% of sensitization.

Mode of Action

The Rh antibodies react with the Rh +ve cells, which have leaked during labour from the foetal circulation to maternal circulation. Thus the process of Anti-D antibody formation in the mother is prevented. 300 mcg neutralizes 15 ml of fetal blood.

Dose and Administration

300 µg Anti-D immunoglobulin is given intramuscularly to the Rh -ve mother within 72 hours after delivery if the baby is Rh +ve (can be given up to 7 days after delivery with some benefit).

Anti-D is given if baby is Rh +ve and the direct Coomb's test is –ve.

Antenatal administration of 300 µg anti-D intramuscularly at 28 weeks reduces the risk of sensitization from 1.2 to 0.2%.

Other Indications

Whenever there is risk of foetomaternal haemorrhage:

1. Abortion–spontaneous or induced: For first trimester abortion, the dose required is 50 µg. In all other conditions, full dose of 300 µg is indicated.
2. Ectopic pregnancy
3. Procedures like chorion villous biopsy, amniocentesis, ECV
4. APH

Kleihauer Test

The test determines the number of foetal cells in maternal circulation. Based on this test, the dose of Anti-D can be decided. 20 µg Anti-D is given per ml of foetal erythrocytes.

When massive foetomaternal haemorrhage is suspected, e.g. caesarean section, manual removal of placenta, additional dose may be required. Routine screening for amount of FMH is advisable as the risk of massive FMH requiring additional anti-D is 1%

ANALGESICS

Pethidine

Dose and administration: 50–100 mg IM

Indications:
1. Pain relief
   - Postoperative
   - During labour
2. Premedication before surgery

Pain Relief in Labour

- To be given during early active phase of labour
- Not to be given when delivery is imminent
- Should not be given in preterm labor
- Should not be given in latent phase of labor as analgesia is unnecessary and sedation may prolong the latent phase.

Side Effects

Nausea, vomiting, respiratory depression of mother and newborn.

Antidote: Naloxone

PROMETHAZINE

This is an antihistaminic agent
Dose and administration: 25 mg IM

Indications

1. In combination with Pethidine to minimize vomiting
2. Premedication
3. Microsurgery for tubal block–perioperative treatment to minimise development of adhesions.

Side effects–sedation

PENTAZOCIN (FORTWIN)

Dose and administration: 30–40 mg IM

Indications

1. Postoperative pain relief
2. Labour analgesia
3. Premedication

METOCLOPRAMIDE
Mode of Action
- Antiemetic agent
- Prevents reflux oesophagitis
- Regularizes GIT motility

Available as
- *Oral:* 10 mg tablets
- *IM:* 5 mg/ml

Indications
1. Hyperemesis gravidarum
2. Reflux oesophagitis–10 mg 8 hourly
3. Before inducing anaesthesia in patients who are not on empty stomach–to prevent aspiration of vomitus (Mendelson's syndrome).

Side Effects
- Sedation
- Extrapyramidal reaction
- Hyperprolactinaemia due to inhibition of pituitary leading to:
  - Galactorrhoea
  - Oligomenorrhoea/amenorrhoea

  Hence, may be given if lactation is inadequate.

VAGINITIS
- Trichomoniasis
- Candidiasis
- Bacterial vaginosis

METRONIDAZOLE
Useful in
- Trichomonial vaginitis
- Bacterial vaginosis

Dose and Administration

Oral dose   *Days*
- 400 mg twice a day   7
- 2 gm   Single dose

For trichomonal vaginitis treatment is given to both partners.

Other Uses

- *Amoebiasis:* 400 mg thrice a day for 5 days
- *Anaerobic infections:* Prophylaxis and treatment 500 mg (100 ml) IV 8 hourly.

Tinidazole or Secnidazole

2 gm single dose may be given for trichomonal vaginitis or bacterial vaginosis.

These drugs are not to be given in first trimester of pregnancy.

Antifungal Agents

Vaginal pessaries are inserted deep inside the vagina at bed time in cases of candidial vaginitis.

Clotrimazole

100 mg vaginal: 1 pessary for 6 days or 200 mg for 3 days. 500 mg single dose vaginally is also useful.

Miconazole

- 200 mg vaginal ovules–1 ovule daily 3 days.
- Cream in the form of 2% gel applied locally

Nystatin

1,00,000 u: 1–2 pessaries for 2 weeks

Fluconazole

150 mg tablet: Single oral dose; not to be given during pregnancy and lactation.

MENORRHAGIA
Drugs Used
- Oestrogen-progestogen combination pills
- Oral progestogens
- Antiprostaglandins
- Danazol
- GnRH analogues (Decapeptyl)
- LNG IUS

Oestrogen-progestogen combination pills are given for 3–6 cycles. They are suitable for young reproductive age group patients.

ORAL PROGESTOGENS
They are suitable for anovular type of dysfunctional uterine bleeding:
- Puberty menorrhagia
- Metropathia haemorrhagica

Drugs
- Norethisterone acetate 5 mg tablet
- Medroxyprogesterone acetate 10 mg tablet.

Dose and Administration
- 10 mg daily for 21 days–from day 5 through day 25
- 10 mg daily in second half of cycle–from day 19 to day 27

Contraindications
- Pregnancy
- Liver dysfunction
- Thromboembolism

MEFENAMIC ACID (ANTIPROSTAGLANDIN)
500 mg tablets three times a day for 5 days during menstruation. Suitable for:
- Painful menorrhagia
- CuT menorrhagia

DANAZOL

200 mg daily for 12 weeks controls menorrhagia. It is not recommended routinely because of its cost and the androgenic side effects.

GnRHa TRIPTORELIN

Injectable depot preparation can be used in menorrhagia when other measures have failed and in cases of myomas before surgery.

LNG IUS

Levonorgestrel releasing intrauterine device is used for contraception and it also relieves menorrhagia.

TREATMENT OF ENDOMETRIOSIS

Combined oral contraceptives, medroxyprogesterone acetate, Danazol, Gestrinone and GnRH agonists can be used for medical management of endometriosis.

DANAZOL

Isoxasole derivative of 17-alfa-ethinyl testosterone. Causes endometrial atrophy, suppresses pituitary and reduces the estrogen-progesterone secretion. Has androgenic and anabolic properties.

Its main use is for tor treatment of endometriosis: 400–800 mg daily for 6 months.

Also can be used for cyclical mastalgia, and fibrocystic disease of breasts.

Side Effects

Weight gain, acne, headache, hirsutism, muscle cramp, breast atrophy, amenorrhoea.

GESTRINONE

Used for treatment of symptoms of endometriosis. It is a 19 norsteroid derivative. Has androgenic, antiestrogenic, antiprogesterone and antipituitary action. Effect similar to Danazol.

Dose

2.5 to 5 mg twice weekly.

Side effects are milder and hence preferred to Danazol.

INDUCTION OF OVULATION

- Clomiphene citrate
- Gonadotropins
- GnRH analogues
- Bromocriptine

CLOMIPHENE CITRATE

It is a nonsteroidal triphenyl ethylene derivative, which is structurally similar to synthetic estrogens diethylstilbestrol (DES). Half-life of the drug is 5–7 days.

Mode of Action

Antioestrogenic action.

Its main action is at the pituitary level via negative feedback in the early follicular phase.

- Interaction with cytoplasmic oestrogen receptors at the cellular level.
- Clomiphene receptor interaction has oestrogen agonist effect in certain organs while oestrogen antagonist effect on other organs.
- The initial rise in FSH is important in initiation of folliculogenesis.
- The resultant increase in plasma oestradiol triggers LH surge. LH surge brings about ovulation.

Indications

- Induction of ovulation in anovulatory infertility in PCOS
- Improving sperm count in certain cases of oligospermia.

Induction of Ovulation

Selection of Cases

- Chronic anovulation due to PCOS
- Presence of adequate endogenous oestrogens is necessary In cases of amenorrhoea, progesterone challenge test should be positive.

Dose and Administration

A. Induction of Ovulation

1. Initially 50 mg daily orally from day 2 to day 6 of menstrual cycle for 5 days.
2. Ovulation monitored by BBT chart, cervical mucus study or ultrasonographic follicle monitoring.
3. If it fails, then the dose may be increased by 50 mg daily in successive cycles. Maximum 150 mg daily.
4. Results:
   - Ovulation rate 70–80%
   - Conception rate 35–40%
5. Reasons for discrepancy in results
   - Corpus luteum defect
   - Hyperprolactinaemia
   - Hyperandrogenism
   - Antioestrogenic effect on cervical mucus
   - Wrong selection of cases
   - Other factors responsible for infertility.

Side Effects

- No serious side effects have been noted so far.
- Multiple pregnancy
- Hot flushes
- Ovarian enlargement and cyst formation; which may lead to rupture and intraperitoneal haemorrhage
- Tinnitus, blurring of vision
- Alopecia, restlessness
- Mild ovarian hyperstimulation can occur
- Increases risk of ovarian malignancy if used for >12 cycles.

Contraindications

- Ovarian failure
- Resistant ovary syndrome
- Non-responsive progesterone challange test
- Ovarian cysts

Clomiphene + Dexamethazone

PCOS with increased levels of DHEAS: 0.5 mg of dexamethazone is given from first to 14th day of cycle. Androgens from adrenals interfering with follicular maturation are suppressed by corticosteroids.

Clomiphene + Oestrogen

Conjugated oestrogens 0.625 mg daily from day 10 through day 16 to increase the quality of cervical mucus which is likely to become poor due to antioestrogenic effect of clomiphene.

Clomiphene + HCG

This combination is indicated where:
- Clomiphene brings about follicular maturation but fails to effect ovulation.
- Ovulation is successfully effected by clomiphene, but subsequently there is corpus luteum deficiency.

Suggested regimes:
5000 to 10000 IU IM when follicle is 18–20 mm. Ovulation occurs 6–40 hours after HCG.

B. *Increasing Sperm Count*

25 mg orally daily for 24 days followed by a gap of one week. Such regime is to be continued for 6 months.

METFORMIN

Used in clomiphene resistant PCOS for ovulation induction 1500 to 2000 mg in two divided doses for 6 months.

Side Effects

GIT upset

BROMOCRIPTINE
Mode of Action
Dopamine agonist
- Reduces levels of prolactin secreted by anterior pituitary.
- May also influence generation of GnRH and other releasing hormones.

Indications
- Infertility with or without amenorrhoea associated with hyperprolactinaemia
- Galactorrhoea with or without amenorrhoea
- *Postpartum:* Chiari-Frommel syndrome
- Idiopathic
- Tumours: Pituitary adenoma, Forbes-Albright syndrome

Dose and Administration
2.5 mg daily in two divided doses for 3–4 days followed by 2.5 mg twice daily.

Monitoring
Galactorrhoea and serum prolactin 4 weekly

The dose is increased if the levels do not decline.

Fall in prolactin levels with resumption of ovulatory cycles is seen usually within 2 months of therapy.

Side Effects
- Nausea
- Headache
- Constipation
- Occasional fainting episodes

Other Uses
- *Inhibition of lactation:* 2.5 mg twice a day for 14 days
- Premenstrual syndrome
- Short luteal phase

- Male hypogonadism
- Acromegaly

CABERGOLINE

Long acting drug, 0.25 mg twice weekly gradually building to 1 mg twice weekly for treatment of hyperprolactinemia. One milligram single dose can be used to suppress lactation in early postpartum period.

GONADOTROPINS

Mode of Action

They act directly on the ovaries to stimulate folliculogenesis.

Indications

- Anovular infertility failing to respond to clomiphene.
- Anovulatory infertility due to hypogonadotropic hypogonadism.
- Stimulation of spermatogenesis in men who have primary or secondary hypogonadotropic hypogonadism.
- Controlled ovarian stimulation in assisted reproduction techniques (ART).

Preparations

- *HMG (Pergonal):* FSH 75 IU + LH 75 IU per ampoule
- *Purified FSH (Metrodin):* FSH 75 IU + very minimal LH activity
- Recombinant FSH is also available
- *HCG:* 1000, 2000 and 5000 IU ampoules.

Administration

The dose of HMG or FSH is titrated as per the individual response, usually guided by ultrasonographic follicle monitoring and serum estradiol (E_2) levels.

Inj. HCG 5000–10000 IU is administered IM when follicle is mature.

Adverse Effects

- Ovarian hyperstimulation
- Increased incidence of multiple pregnancy
- Ovarian enlargement with multiple cyst formation, haemoconcentration and tendency for thrombosis.
- Ovary(ies) may become tense and friable and vulnerable for rupture with trivial stimulus like coitus or abdominal palpation. This may lead to severe internal haemorrhage. In milder cases, patient will present with abdominal pain, nausea, distention of abdomen and ascites.

Disadvantages

i. Requires laboratory monitoring
ii. Requires highly expert infertologist
iii. Increased risk of multiple pregnancy
iv. Increased incidence of abortion
v. Highly expensive treatment.

GnRH ANALOGUES (GnRHa)

Indications

Ovulation induction in controlled ovarian hyperstimulation protocols for ART.

Mode of Action

Profound LH and FSH suppression:
- Competitive binding with GnRH receptors
- Down regulation of GnRH receptors.

Preparations

- Leuprolide acetate subcutaneous injections daily
- Nafarelin acetate (intranasally, once daily).

Administration

Can be started from midluteal phase of previous cycle. HMG is started when serum E_2 is sufficiently low. GnRHa and HMG continued with follicle monitoring until HCG administration.

Alternatively

HMG and GnRHa can be started simultaneously from day 2 and continued up to HCG administration.

PULSATILE GnRH AGONIST THERAPY

Indications

Induction of ovulation in hypothalamic failure.

Method of Administration

GnRH is administered in 2 hourly IV dosage by a special automatic syringe which delivers predetermined volumes of the drug at set intervals. This effects pulsatile administration of GnRH mimicking natural pulsatile release from hypothalamus.

Advantages

  i. More physiological
 ii. Ovarian hyperstimulation syndrome rare
iii. No need for expensive monitoring.

Other Uses

1. GnRH stimulation test for differential diagnosis of primary and secondary amenorrhoea.
2. Differencial diagnosis of hypogonadism in men and women.
3. Initiating puberty and sexual development in males and females with isolated idiopathic hypogonadotropic hypogonadism.

GnRH Agonists Depot Forms: Triptorelin (Decapeptyl)

- To shrink the uterine myomas and control menorrhagia 3.75 mg depot injections every 28 days for 3 cycles. Myomas usually regrow after cessation of therapy
- Endometriosis
- Menorrhagia if other treatment fails
- Precocious puberty

Expensive

Side effects: Menopausal symptoms, osteoporosis if treatment continued for >6 months.

Cetrorelix (GnRH antagonist)

Gonadotropin-releasing hormone (GnRH) antagonists have been introduced in clinical practice for controlled ovarian hyperstimulation in ART cycles. Because GnRH antagonists competitively bind to pituitary GnRH receptors, they directly and rapidly inhibit gonadotropin release within several hours. GnRH antagonists can be used to prevent a surge of luteinizing hormone during controlled ovarian hyperstimulation for assisted conception. They give similar live-birth rates as GnRH agonists but with markedly lower incidence of severe ovarian hyperstimulation syndrome (OHSS).

HORMONES

OESTROGENS

Preparations available

1. Ethinyl estradiol	Lynoral 0.01 mg, 0.05 mg
2. Oestriol	Evalon 1 mg, 2 mg
	Evalon vaginal cream 1 mg/gm
3. Conjugated equine estrogens	Premarin, conjugase 0.625 mg tablet daily
4. Oestradiol–estraderm TTS	25 μg, 50 μg, 100 μg transdermal patches
5. 17 β-estradiol gel 0.06%	1.5 mg daily transdermal application

Clinical Uses

1. Hormone replacement therapy for:
   - Menopausal vasomotor symptoms
   - Prevention of osteoporosis
   - Atrophic vaginitis–estrogen vaginal cream used
   - Genitourinary symptoms of menopause

2. Oestrogen–progesterone challenge test for the evaluation of primary and secondary amenorrhoea
3. Development of secondary sexual characteristics in primary gonadal failure
4. DUB–threshold bleeding
5. Hormonal contraception: Combined oral pills/injections
6. Vulvovaginitis in prepubertal girls
7. Labial adhesions
8. Ashermann's syndrome–after lysis of synechiae
9. Treatment of hirsutism

Contraindications
Absolute

- History of thromboembolic disorders
- Cholestasis
- Liver dysfunction
- Breast cancer
- Pregnancy/lactation

Relative

- Hypertension
- Diabetes mellitus
- Epilepsy
- Migraine

Side Effects

- Nausea
- Vomiting
- Mastalgia
- Oedema
- Weight gain

Long-term use in postmenopausal women: Risk of endometrial hyperplasia and endometrial carcinoma.

PROGESTERONES

Progestogens for Use in Gynaecologic Conditions

1. Medroxyprogesterone acetate	10 mg, 2.5 mg tablets
2. Norethisterone	5 mg tablets
3. Norgestrel in combined OC pills	
4. Lynestrenol	5 mg tablets
5. Dydrogesterone	5 mg tablets

Clinical Uses

1. *Contraception:* Combined oral pills, progesterone only contraception (injections, minipills, implants, LNG IUS)
2. Endometriosis
3. Menorrhagia–anovular dysfunctional uterine bleeding
4. Progesterone challenge test in evaluation of amenorrhoea
5. Endometrial hyperplasia
6. Advanced endometrial carcinoma–palliative management
7. Hormone replacement therapy–along with oestrogens to minimise the effect of oestrogens on endometrium
8. Precocious puberty

Contraindications

- Breast cancer
- Genital cancer
- Liver disease
- Pregnancy

Progestogens for Use in Pregnancy

1. Allylestranol	5 mg tablets
2. Hydroxyprogesterone caproate	250 mg/ml, 500 mg/ml IM
3. Natural micronized progesterone	100 mg, 200 mg tablets oral/vaginal
4. Dydrogesterone	5 mg tablets

These preparations are used in for prevention of early miscarriages and prevention of preterm labour.

HORMONE REPLACEMENT THERAPY (HRT) FOR MENOPAUSE
Indications
- To relieve symptoms of menopause (hot flashes, genitourinary, psychological symptoms)
- To reduce the risk of osteoporosis.
- To maintain the individual's well-being.

Contraindications
- Known/suspected breast or endometrial cancer
- Undiagnosed abnormal genital bleeding
- Active thromboembolic disorders
- Active liver or gallbladder disease
- *Relative contraindications:* Heart disease, migrainous headaches, H/O liver/gallbladder disease

For hysterectomized women only estrogen replacement is necessary. There is no need for progesterone.

For women having uterus: Combination estrogen + progestin therapy is recommended. To prevent estrogen induced endometrial hyperplasia, progestogens are given for 12–14 days of each month or in a continuous combined manner.

Routes of Administration
Oral, nonoral (vaginal, transdermal, subcutaneous implants).

Oral
Conjugated estrogens 0.3 mg to 0.625 mg daily
    Medroxyprogesterone acetate (MPA) 10 mg daily for 12–14 days or 2.5 mg daily continuously.

Problems
- Irregular and unpredictable uterine bleeding is common. This needs evaluation in a postmenopausal lady.
- Risk of breast cancer and thromboembolism is increased with longer duration of use.
- Lowest effective dose should be used for shortest duration.

- With short-term therapy up to 5 years, risks are not increased
- Diet, lifestyle adaptation is important
- Annual review is necessary

Transdermal Estrogen Patch

0.025 mg every 4 days (twice weekly) continuous non-cyclic therapy may be indicated in hysterectomized women. Cyclical administration is recommended (21 days of therapy with 7 days gap). In women with an intact uterus, a progestin should be sequentially administered for 12 to 14 days per cycle to avoid overstimulation of endometrium.

Advantage

Hepatic first-pass effect not seen with non-oral HRT. No effect on coagulation factors.

Decreases serum triglycerides. Suitable for women having hypertriglyceridemia.

TIBOLONE

- Gonadomimetic steroid
- Estrogenic, progestogenic and week androgenic action
- Used for HRT in menopausal women. To be started one year after menopause
- 2.5 mg daily continuously
- No risk of endometrial proliferation (bleed free HRT).

NONHORMONAL THERAPY FOR MENOPAUSAL WOMEN

ALENDRONATE

Bisphosphonate
- Used for protection from postmenopausal osteoporosis
- Inhibits osteoclastic activity, prevents bone loss associated with estrogen 2 deprivation
- Dose: 35–70 mg/weekly orally
- To be taken on empty stomach with large glass of water, remain upright for 30–60 min.

RALOXIFENE

Selective estrogen receptor modulator
Dose: 60 mg/day
- Nonhormonal therapy for preventing bone loss
- Estrogen like action on bone and lipids without stimulating the breast or endometrium. Decreased vertebral fractures, reduced risk of breast cancer
- No endometrial stimulation (Tamoxifen acts as estrogen agonist in the endometrum increasing the risk of endometrial polyps, hyperplasia, cancer)
- *Side effects:* Leg cramps
- Increased vasomotor symptoms
- *Potential risks:* Venous thromboembolic events increased.

Other therapies for menopausal symptoms:
- Soy, isoflavones 100 mg/day
- Vit E 800 IU/day
- Pyridoxine
- Clonidine can be given for hot flashes if estrogens are contraindicated.

HIRSUTISM

Combined oral contraceptive pills specially those containing cyproterone acetate are used.

Spironolactone, ketoconazole, flutamide and finasteride can be used.

SPIRONOLACTONE

Potassium sparing diuretic. It has antiandrogenic effect and is used in treatment of hirsutism (100–150 mg daily along with cyclical estrogens). It can cause feminization of male fetus if given during pregnancy.

CHEMOTHERAPY IN GYNAECOLOGICAL MALIGNANCIES

GESTATIONAL TROPHOBLASTIC DISEASES

Single agent therapy by Methotrexate or Actinomycin D can be given to postmolar gestational trophoblastic neoplasia and low risk choriocarcinoma.

METHOTREXATE

Mode of Action

Antimetabolite agent.

Dose and Administration

50 mg (1 mg/kg body weight) IV on alternate days for 4 days (days 1, 3, 5 and 7).

Injection Folinic acid 6 mg IM 24 hours after each Methotrexate injection.

Methotrexate 50 mg/m^2 body surface area can be given weekly also.

Side Effects

- Stomatitis
- Myelosuppression
- Liver toxicity
- Renal toxicity

Other Uses

1. Medical management of ectopic pregnancy
2. Placenta accreta–small remnants of placental bits
3. Abdominal pregnancy–remnants of placental tissue that could not be surgically removed and had to be left behind.

ACTINOMYCIN D

This is an antibiotic.

Dose and Administration

10–12 µg/kg/day for 5 days

Adverse Effects

- Nausea
- Vomiting
- Diarrhoea
- Bone marrow depression

Multiple agents therapy by following regimes is recommended for high risk choriocarcinoma.

MAC: Methotrexate + Actinomycin D + Cyclophosphamide

EMA–CO: Etoposide + Methotrexate + Vincristine + Actinomycin D + Cyclophosphamide.

OVARIAN CANCER

High grade, high risk stage I a and b, stage I c and all advanced ovarian cancer cases should be treated by combination chemotherapy or at least single agent chemotherapy.

CYCLOPHOSPHAMIDE

This is an alkylating agent used for many years.

500–1000 mg/m^2 IV to be repeated every 3 weeks for about 6 cycles.

Adverse Effects

- Nausea
- Vomiting
- Alopecia
- Bone marrow depression

CISPLATINUM

75 mg/m^2 IV infusion to be repeated every 3 weeks.

Adverse Effects

- Nausea
- Vomiting
- Nephrotoxicity
- Ototoxicity
- Neurotoxicity
- Bone marrow depression

Combination of cisplatinum and cyclophosphamide is found to be effective in epithelial ovarian malignancy.

Carboplatin given IV has less nephrotoxicity, neurotoxicity and ototoxicity than cisplatinum and is preferred although it is more expensive and has more mylosuppressive effect. The dose is calculated by a special formula taking into consideration the GFR and may range between 350 and 450 mg.

Paclitaxel is the drug of choice for advanced ovarian cancer as single agent or in combination with carboplatin.

Dose 135 to175 mg/m^2 every 3 weeks for 6 cycles

Other agents used: Doxorubicin, Topotecan, Etoposide, Docetaxel.

Cisplatinum is also used in combined chemoradiation therapy for endometrial carcinoma and for carcinoma cervix specially recurrent and advanced cancer cases.

ANTIRETROVIRAL THERAPY (ART) DURING PREGNANCY

Over 90% of HIV infection in children is acquired by transmission from infected mothers to their infants. The transmission occurs maximally in perinatal period. Postnatal transmission takes place mainly through breast milk.

General Principles for ART during Pregnancy

1. All HIV infected pregnant women should be offered ART to reduce risk of mother to child transmission (MTCT) of HIV.
2. Combination antiretroviral (ARV) regimes are more effective than single ARV regimes.
3. Longer duration of ART administration during pregnancy reduces antepartum and intrapartum transmission more effectively as compared to short protocols.
4. Exposed newborn should receive prophylactic ART for 4–6 weeks.
5. HIV infected woman who has not received any ART during pregnancy and seen in labor should receive intrapartum ART.
6. Infants born to HIV infected women who have not received antenatal or intrapartum ART should receive ART.
7. If patient is on ART before gestation, it should be continued during pregnancy. Efavirenze should be avoided in first trimester. Zidovudine (AZT) should be one of the drugs during pregnancy to prevent MTCT.

8. Potential adverse effects on placental function and fetus/ newborn should be discussed with patients.

PPTCT PROGRAM

Under National Prevention of Parent to Child Transmission (PPTCT) of HIV program, every pregnant woman is counseled to undergo HIV test and all consenting women are tested for HIV during pregnancy. Women testing negative are offered post test counseling and are encouraged to stay negative by following safe sex. Those testing positive are counseled regarding strategies for preventing transmission of HIV infection to their babies and regarding care for their own health.

ART for maternal health: HIV positive women have their complete clinical examination and have their CD4 count done. Women having CD4 count <350 need ART for their own health hence they are referred to ART centre for initiation of 3 drug therapy (HAART). All WHO clinical stage III & IV and those having CD4 count <350 are eligible for ART for their own health. ART should be started irrespective of gestational age and continued throughout life. One regime of first line drugs include AZT, Lamivudine (3TC) and Nevirapine. Careful monitoring is necessary to monitor the side effects and major adverse effects of drugs. Baby should receive prophylactic ART for 4–6 weeks.

Prophylactic ART: The women who do not need ART for their own health are given prophylactic ART to prevent transmission of HIV to their baby.

There are various regimes of different drug combinations administered to pregnant mother during pregnancy and labour. Prophylactic ART is administered to the newborn baby also. Landmark studies guiding the therapy are:
- ACTG 076 protocol
  - *Antenatal (after 14 weeks):* AZT 300 mg orally twice a day until onset of labour
  - *Intranatal:* AZT IV infusion or 300 mg orally at the onset of labor and every 3 hours thereafter until delivery
  - *Infant:* AZT 2 mg/kg/6 hours orally for 6 weeks, beginning 8 to 12 hours afterbirth.

Relative efficacy is 68% (infection status at age 18 months in non-breastfed babies)

- CDC/Thai regime
  - Antenatal AZT 300 mg orally BD from 36 weeks till onset of labor
  - Intranatal AZT 300 mg orally every 3 hours
  - *Infant (newborn):* None (no breastfeeding).

  Relative efficacy is 50% (infection status at age 6 months)

- HIVNET 012 protocol: Administration of single dose nevirapine (sd NVP) to both mother and the newborn. This is made available in the National PPTCT Program.
  - *Mother:* Nevirapine 200 mg orally single dose at the onset of labor
  - *Infant:* Nevirapine 2 mg/kg orally as single dose administered within 72 hours of birth.

  Relative efficacy is 47% (infection status at age 14 weeks in predominantly breastfed babies).

  The WHO guidelines (2010) recommend the following ART regimes for mother and the newborn baby for different case scenarios.

I. Mother Reporting in Pregnancy, no Indication for ARV Treatment

AZT 300 mg BD daily orally during pregnancy from 14 weeks onwards till onset of labor and 3 hourly during labor.

(If mother has received AZT for <4 weeks, additional therapy by 3TC and sd NVP is recommended during labour and continuing AZT and 3TC for 7 days after delivery) alternatively.

Maternal triple ARV: More effective reduction in viral load: AZT/3TC/NVP from 14 weeks onwards, continued through labor

Infant is given syrup AZT

Transmission risk is significantly reduced to <1%

Limitations: Costly regime, adverse effects of ARVs

II. Mother Reporting in Labour, not Received ARV

Intrapartum: AZT + 3TC + sd NVP
Postpartum: Continue AZT + 3TC for 7 days to mother to prevent NVP resistance mutations
Infant: sd NVP + AZT 4 weeks

III. Mother has not Received ARV and is Delivered

Single dose NVP as soon as possible to baby and AZT for 4 weeks
Alternatively
Sd NVP + AZT for 1 week
Both more effective than sd NVP alone
AZT given to infant reduces risk of NVP resistance if baby gets infected.

For reducing breast milk transmissions while retaining the advantages of breastfeeding specially in resource poor settings, various studies have used ARV during postnatal period to breastfeeding mother or infant. Continuing maternal triple ARV regime until one week after complete cessation of breastfeeding is recommended. Administration of extended Nevirapine to the infant has also been studied.

Prophylactic ART regimes given to mother do not benefit the mother. They are administered to reduce the risk of vertical transmission.

Safety of ARV

AZT and Nevirapine have favorable safety profile for infants. No other ARV is recommended to exposed infants. AZT anemia is reversible after discontinuing the drug.

For mothers AZT, 3 TC or FTC, and Nevirapine have favorable safety profile.

- AZT has risk of anemia and neutropenia.
- Nevirapine has risk of severe rash and liver toxicity and is not recommended for women with higher CD4 count because of higher toxicity risk in this group.
- Efavirenze is not recommended in first trimester of pregnancy for fear of teratogenicity (recent studies have

shown that it does not increase this risk). There is risk of rash and neuropsychiatric problems also.

- 3TC is generally safe however there is concern of hepatitis B flare if mother is HBV-coinfected and drug is stopped.

While on therapy, monitor hemoglobin, WBC, platelet count, liver enzymes and serum creatinine periodically.

Newborn: Complete blood count is monitored.

Drug resistance: So far short course of AZT during pregnancy has not been shown to result in drug resistance and the benefits clearly outweigh the risks.

Maternal single dose nevirapine: Resistant mutations reported in many studies. Long half-life NVP is responsible. Resistance however diminishes over time. AZT/3TC 'Tail' for 7 days postpartum has been shown to result in significant reduction in NVP resistance.

Terratogenic Drugs

Drugs that Affect the Foetus

Drug	Effect
ACE inhibitors	Neonatal renal failure
Alcohol	Foetal alcohol syndrome, Micro-cephaly, Mental retardation, Craniofacial dysmorphism, developmental delay
Antithyroid	Foetal goiter, cretinism, mental retardation
Caffeine	Increased abortion and stillbirth rate
Chloramphenicol	Gray baby syndrome
Ganglion blocking agents	Neonatal paralytic ileus
Long acting sulfonmides, Trimethoprim, Salicylates, Phenothiazines	Neonatal jaundice and kernicterus
Nicotine	IUGR
Oral antidiabetic agents	Abnormalities of eyes, CNS, skeletal system, neonatal hypoglycaemia
Streptomycin, kanamycin, gentamycin	Congenital deafness due to action on 8th cranial nerve
Tetracycline	Stains teeth and bones by chealating calcium

Warfarin	Cerebral haemorrhage, nasal hypo-plasia, ophthalmic abnormalities, microcephaly, mental retardation

Drugs that Affect the Embryo

Drug	Effect
Androgens, synthetic progestogens	Masculinization of female foetus
Anticonvulsants	Congenital heart disease, cleft palate, microcephaly, facial dysmorphism
Corticosteroids	Cleft palate, cleft lip
Cytotoxic Drugs	Abortion, multiple malformations
Diethylstilbestrol	Vaginal adenosis/adenocarcinoma in females in adolescence
Thalidomide	Phocomelia, cardiac malformations

Effects of Drugs on Neonate during Lactation

Drug	Effect
Anticoagulants	Haemorrhage tendency
Antihistaminics	Drowsiness
Antimetabolites	Anti-DNA activity, immunosuppressant
Antithyroids	Hypothyroidism and goiter
Bromides	Bromism, rash, drowsiness, lethargy and poor feeding
Chloramphenicol	Bone marrow toxicity Gray baby syndrome
Diazepam, opiates, phenobarbitone	Sedative' poor suckling reflex
Isoniazide	Anti-DNA activity Hepatotoxicity
Oral pills	Suppression of lactation
Tetracycline	Colouring of teeth, chelation of Ca^{++} in bones and teeth

Instruments in Obstetrics and Gynaecology

31. Opening Abdomen
32. Instruments

Opening Abdomen

By and large, a gynaecological surgeon has to restrict his surgery to the pelvic organs, though his approach to them may be abdominal or pelvic. During abdominal surgery, he enters the abdomen by an incision in subumbilical–hypogastric region. There are different incisions to open the abdomen.

The choice of incision is influenced by a number of factors:
- Adequate operative exposure
- Pelvic pathology for which surgery is being performed
- Simplicity and speed of the operation
- Presence of previous scar
- Presence of incisional hernia
- Abdominal contour
- Cosmetic consideration
- Strength of healing scar
- Postoperative comfort of the patient.

The following layers of anterior abdominal wall are opened:
- Skin
- Superficial fascia
- Deep or Scarpa's fascia
- Anterior rectus sheath
- Recti (and sometimes external oblique) muscles
- Posterior rectus sheath with transversalis fascia
- Parietal peritoneum.

While incising the parietal peritoneum, care should be taken to avoid injury to the intra-abdominal organs like intestines, urinary bladder, omentum, etc. Picking up the peritoneum at a higher level in two nontraumatising tissue forceps, palpating the picked up fold of peritoneum to confirm the absence of any other tissue in it and then only incising by blade of a scalpel is the safest way to avoid any injury to the deeper structures. The nick taken then should be extended under vision by a pair of scissors with two fingers under it to protect the viscera.

The different types of incisions for opening the abdomen through anterior abdominal wall are:

A. Vertical incisions
　1. Midline incision
　2. Paramedian incision
B. Transverse incisions
　1. Pfannenstiel incision
　2. Joel Cohen incision
　3. Transverse muscle cutting incision (Maylard)
　4. Cherney incision

A. Vertical Incisions

Midline Incision

- The skin is incised in the midline in the subumbilical area.
- Superficial fascia and deep fascia are dissected. Proper haemostasis is achieved during this step.
- Rectus sheath is picked up in tissue forceps and a nick is taken in it by scalpel blade. The incision is extended vertically cranially and caudally towards the symphysis pubis by a pair of scissors.
- The two recti are separated from each other to expose the anterior parietal peritoneum.
- Parietal peritoneum is opened as explained above.

Advantages

- Midline being less vascular, bleeding is less.
- Quicker way of entering the abdomen.
- No risk of injuring any important structure.
- Good exposure on both sides.

Disadvantages

- Incidence of incisional hernia more (recent studies however have shown little difference in dehiscence rates between properly closed midline incisions and transverse incisions)

- If the incision is to be extended cranially, it has to be done around the umbilicus; otherwise, the umbilicus has to be removed.
- Intestines encroach in the field of operation.

Paramedian Incision

The skin and rectus sheath are incised vertically about one inch lateral to the midline on either side. The rectus muscle is dissected from the rectus sheath medially to reach midline. Both recti are separated from each other to expose anterior parietal peritoneum, which is opened vertically in midline.

Advantages
- The incidence of burst abdomen is less
- Less incidence of incisional hernia
- No difficulty in extending the incision above
- Good exposure of abdomen and pelvis
- Healing is good.

Disadvantage
Paramedian region being more vascular, there is more bleeding and more time is spent in achieving haemostasis. However, with the use of bipolar cautery this can be minimised.

B. Transverse Incisions

Pfannenstiel Incision

It is transverse incision, which is slightly curved with concavity upward at its lateral ends. The incision is usually made 2–3 cm (2 finger breadths) above the pubic crest. Usually it extends about 10–15 cm in length.

- The skin is incised in the manner mentioned above.
- Subcutaneous fascia is dissected simultaneously ensuring the haemostasis to reach the rectus sheath.
- Rectus sheath is incised transversely, taking care not to injure the branches of epigastric vessels at its lateral end.
- The cut edges of rectus sheath are separated from underlying rectus muscles on either side.
- Two recti are separated from each other.
- Anterior parietal peritoneum is opened vertically.

Advantages
- Risk of incisional hernia is reduced
- Less postoperative discomfort to the patient
- Cosmetic advantage due to hidden scar
- Easy to keep intestines away during surgery

Disadvantages
- More time required for opening and closure
- Increased operative bleeding
- Lesser exposure than midline incision. Not suitable for surgical staging of gynecological tumors
- Intestinal surgery not possible
- Not suitable for large pelvic tumours
- Risk of damage to ilioinguinal and iliohypogastric nerves supplying the mons pubis.

Since inferior epigastric vessels may be encountered in the lateral margin of the incision, if proper haemostatic care is not taken, bleeding may occur.

Joel Cohen Incision

This is a straight transverse incision, 3 cm below a line that joins both anterior superior iliac spines. Subsequent tissue layers are opened bluntly and, if necessary, extended with scissors and not knife. This incision is used in caesarean section operation by Misgav Ladach technique. It is associated with less postoperative pain, less requirement for analgesia and minimal postoperative febrile morbidity.

Transverse Muscle Cutting Incision (Maylard incision)

This incision gives better exposure required for the ultramajor pelvic surgery.
- For Gynec surgery, the skin and rectus sheath are incised transversely similar to Pfannenstiel incision
- Identification and severing the inferior epigastric vessels between the ligations is important to avoid the retraction and haematoma formation in the lateral margins of incision.
- After ligation of the inferior epigastric vessels, electrocautery is used to transversely cut the rectus muscle.

- The peritoneum is opened transversely

In closing this incision, it is preferable to include the fascia with each stitch while suturing the muscle so as to avoid cutting through the muscles, Polyglactin (Vicryl) suture no. 1 is used for this purpose.

Advantages
- Excellent exposure
- Since the nerves and blood vessels enter the abdominal wall muscles in the same direction as the incision, they are not severed. Therefore, anatomically, this incision produces a strong scar.
- Incision does not cut across the nerve endings excessively nor does it devitalise segments of the abdominal wall.

Disadvantages
- More time required for incising and reapproximating the abdominal muscles.
- Risk of potential injury to the ilioinguinal, iliohypogastric and femoral nerves.

Cherney Incision

This is a transverse incision that allows excellent surgical exposure to the space of Retzius and the pelvic sidewall. Generally, it is used for modified Burch colposuspension for stress urinary incontinence.

The skin and fascia are cut in a manner similar to a Maylard incision. The rectus muscles are separated to the pubic symphysis and separated from the pyramidalis muscles. Using electrocautery, the rectus tendons are cut from the pubic bone. The rectus muscles are retracted and the peritoneum opened. While closing the abdomen, the cut ends of the rectus muscle are attached to the distal end of the anterior rectus sheath with interrupted nonabsorbable sutures.

Closure of Abdomen

The peritoneum does not need closure as re-epithelization occurs within 48 hours and it does not add strength to the incision.

The fascia is approximated with a continuous running suture using delayed absorbable suture, this is faster. The dehiscence rates are comparable to those of interrupted closures. Alternatively, interrupted Smead-Jones (far-far, near-near suturing) technique may be used.

Routine closure of the subcutaneous tissue space should not be used, unless the woman has more than 2 cm subcutaneous fat, because it does not reduce the incidence of wound infection.

32

Instruments

VAGINAL SPECULAE

These instruments are used for visualizing vagina and cervix for diagnostic and therapeutic purposes.

1. Sim's Speculum

It is double ended speculum with blades of different sizes at both the ends.

Uses

For retracting posterior vaginal wall for:

a. Examination of genital prolapse

b. Vaginal surgery

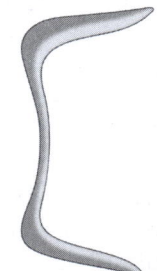

Advantage

Good exposure of vagina and cervix is obtained.

Fig. 32.1: Sim's speculum

Disadvantages

i. An assistant is required to hold the speculum.

ii. Anterior vaginal wall retractor is required for proper exposure of cervix and vagina.

iii. Patient has to be taken to the edge of the examination table. Alternatively, the patient is made to lie in Sim's position, i.e. left lateral position. It is unsuitable for routine OPD use.

Method of Introduction

Labia are separated by left hand and the blade of the speculum is introduced in anteroposterior diameter of the vagina. Then the blade is gently rotated in 90°.

2. Cusco's Bivalve Self-retaining Vaginal Speculum

It has got two hinged blades, which can be opened inside the vagina. The blades can be held in open position with the help of a screw.

Uses

a. To inspect the cervix and vagina for any lesions
b. For collecting vaginal discharge for microbiological studies
c. For collecting material from cervix and vagina for cytological study.

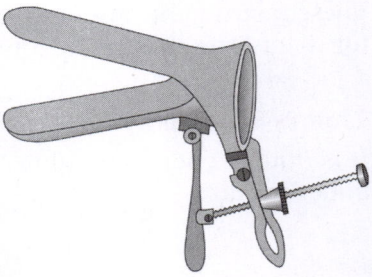

Fig. 32.2: Cusco's speculum

Advantages

i. Assistant is not required
ii. Patient can be examined in dorsal position without taking her to the edge of the table.
iii. Suitable for use in out patient clinic.

Disadvantage

Unsuitable for use in vaginal surgical procedures.

3. Auvard's Speculum

This is a very heavy speculum with a single curved blade and a long grooved handle, on which a detachable lead ball is fitted. The instrument weighs about 2.0 kg.

Advantages

• No assistant is required to hold the speculum in place as due to the weight of the instrument and angle of the blade, it remains in position.

- Good exposure in vagina
- Very convenient during vaginal operations.

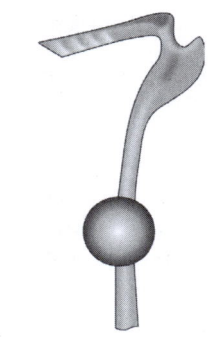

Disadvantage

It is very painful to tolerate the weight of the speculum in vagina. Therefore, this instrument has to be used only when the patient is properly anaesthetised and is in lithotomy position.

Fig. 32.3: Auvard's speculum

4. Soonawala Speculum

This 'Z' shaped speculum has got two blades of different sizes with a weight attached to its shank.

Advantages

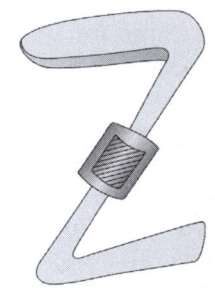

- No assistant is required to hold it in place.
- Was found suitable for mass vaginal sterilization camps conducted in past?

Initially smaller blade is used and after opening the pouch of Douglas, the longer blade is introduced.

Fig. 32.4: Soonawala speculum

Sim's Anterior Vaginal Wall Retractor

This is a long stout instrument having angulated ends. Both the loops are having fenestrations and horizontal serrations on them.

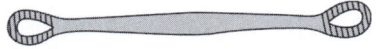

Fig. 32.5: Sim's anterior vaginal wall retractor

Use

This instrument is used along with Sim's speculum for inspecting cervix and vagina by retracting anterior vaginal wall.

Jayle's Vaginal Retractor

This self-retaining vaginal lateral wall retractor is used during vaginal surgery. It has one fixed blade while the other is sliding. A screw is provided for sliding adjustment. It gives a good exposure and minimises the need of an assistant.

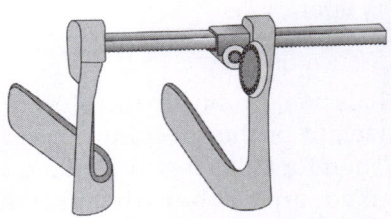

Fig. 32.6: Jayle's retractor

Comyns-Berkeley's Vulval Retractor

It has got two adjustable blades with hooked pointed ends. The blades can be opened and adjusted by a screw. It is used for retracting labia in operations on vulva. There are varieties of vulval retractors. They have hooks to retract labia and adjustment screw to hold the retracted ends in their position. Vulval stay sutures can be used instead of retractor.

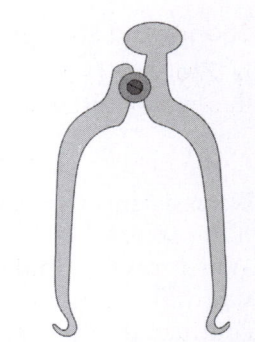

Fig. 32.7: Comyns-Berkeley's vulval retractor

INSTRUMENTS FOR GRASPING AND STEADYING CERVIX

1. Volsellum Forceps

This is a long instrument curved on flat having sharp teeth at its working end and a catch at the handle which gives a firm grip of the cervix.

During its use the curvature of the instrument should face anteriorly to negotiate the angle of vagina. A firm grip of the cervical lip should be obtained; otherwise slipping of the

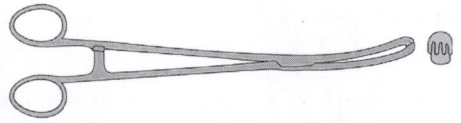

Fig. 32.8: Volsellum forceps

instrument can damage the cervix considerably, with risk of subsequent infection.

Uses

a. To hold anterior lip of the cervix in gynaecological vaginal operations like D & C, cervical biopsy, cauterization of cervix, insertion of intrauterine contraceptive device, etc.
b. To catch posterior the lip of cervix for:
   • Posterior colpopuncture (culdocentesis) in suspected ruptured ectopic pregnancy
   • Posterior colpotomy for drainage of pelvic abscess
   • Examination of enterocoele in genital prolapse
   • Culdoscopy and vaginal sterilization.

2. Tenaculum Forceps

It is a long straight instrument having one sharp point on each jaw in the plane of the handle and a catch at the handle. It has no curvature.

Advantage

Being a straight instrument a steady traction can be given on the cervix to ensure a leak proof fitting of the tubal patency cannula.

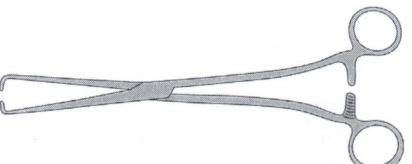

Fig. 32.9: Tenaculum forceps

Use

For holding cervix while performing tubal patency tests, hydrotubation, etc.

The instrument is applied horizontally to both the anterior and posterior cervical lips. They should not encroach on the cervical os, thus allowing the tubal patency cannula to fit snugly over the external os.

3. Sponge Holding Forceps

During pregnancy, the cervix is very soft and highly vascular. instruments like volsellum or tenaculum forceps having pointed jaws may injure such a cervix; hence this nontraumatic instrument is used to hold the cervix in following conditions:

a. Evacuation in cases of incomplete abortions
b. Cervical encerclage
c. To explore the cervix for excluding cervical tears
d. While suturing cervical tears, following delivery or abortions

INSTRUMENTS USED FOR DISINFECTING THE PARTS

1. Sponge Holding Forceps

This instrument is designed for holding swabs to apply antiseptic lotions to different parts. It is a long instrument with fenestrated serrated blades and a catch at the handle.

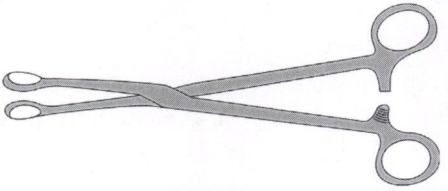

Fig. 32.10: Sponge holding forceps

Uses

a. Application of antiseptic lotions while painting the parts prior to surgical procedures.
b. Holding sponges for applying pressure on deep bleeding points.
c. Holding cervix in obstetrical conditions.
d. Pushing the bladder away from the uterus during abdominal hysterectomy.
e. Compressing infundibulopelvic ligaments temporarily to minimise operative bleeding during myomectomy.
f. Holding the edges of the lower uterine segment during caesarean section where Green-Armytage forceps are not available. Care should be taken to avoid passing the needle through the fenestration of the instrument.
g. Removing the products of conception where ovum forceps are not available. Care should be taken not to use the catch of the instrument.

2. Playfair's Probe

This long straight instrument with rounded tip has spiked roughened end to hold cotton around it. A thin film of cotton is wrapped firmly around the spiked rough surface which is dipped in dilute iodine. The tip of the instrument is introduced through the cervical canal and rotated to disinfect cervical canal.

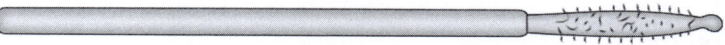

Fig. 32.11: Playfair's probe

Use

To disinfect the cervical canal before introducing any instrument into the uterine cavity.

SOUNDS

1. Uterine Sound

This is a long instrument with 45° angulation 2.5 inches from its tip to negotiate the uterine flexion. It has got markings throughout its length.

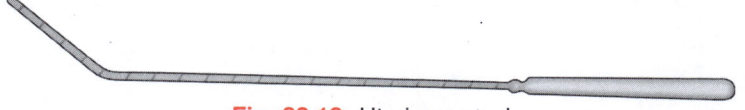

Fig. 32.12: Uterine sound

Uses

a. To measure the length of the uterus and to confirm its position as a preliminary step in procedures like IUD insertions, D & C, etc.

b. In cases of missing threads of IUD:
   During plain X-ray of the uterus in anteroposterior and lateral views, sound is inserted in the uterine cavity to demarcate the position of the uterine cavity. This helps in knowing the position of IUD in relation to the uterine cavity.

c. To note the extent of elongation of cervix in cases of genital prolapse.

d. Irregularity in the uterine cavity can be detected which arouses the suspicion of submucous myoma or developmental anomalies of uterus.

e. Differentiating cervical polyp from chronic inversion of uterus.

It should not be used in pregnancy and in presence of lower genital tract infection.

2. Bladder Sound

The terminal portion of bladder sound is smoothly curved. The instrument does not have markings.

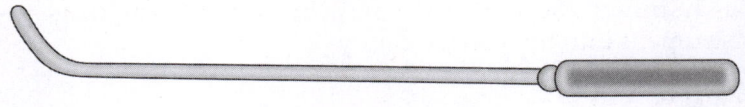

Fig. 32.13: Bladder sound

Uses

a. This instrument has been devised for sounding a calculus in the bladder.

b. To note the extent of cystocele during anterior colporrhaphy

c. To note the level of bladder in vaginal hysterectomy before opening the anterior peritoneal pouch.

d. To differentiate cystocoele from anterior vaginal wall cyst.

INSTRUMENTS FOR DILATING CERVIX

Metal dilators are used for rapid dilatation of cervix while laminaria or isapgol tents effect slow painless dilatation of cervix.

1. Hegar's Dilators

These are usually double ended; however, single ended Hegar's dilators are also available. They are slightly curved at the ends and have a uniform diameter throughout their length. They are graduated by 1 mm. Number of the dilator indicates its diameter in mm.

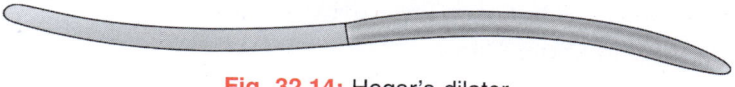

Fig. 32.14: Hegar's dilator

2. Fenton's Dilators

These are double ended dilators with a marked curve for the uterine flexion. These are gradual dilators having maximum thickness proximally and tapering end. Usually, the sizes graduate from the tip to the maximum diameter by three mm.

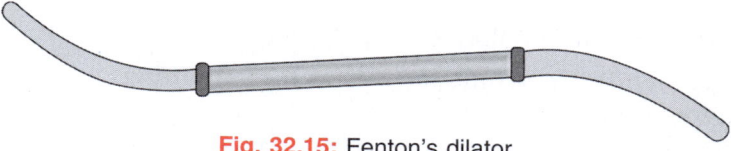

Fig. 32.15: Fenton's dilator

3. Purandare's Dilators

They come in a set of four. They are single ended dilators with shoulders. They are having three graduations in each dilator making the dilatation easy with minimum trauma to the cervix. Also due to shoulders risk of perforation is reduced. Hence, they are more suitable in suction evacuation.

4. Denniston Dilators

These are light weight plastic dilators. They are available in set of five. These can be sterilized even by autoclaving.

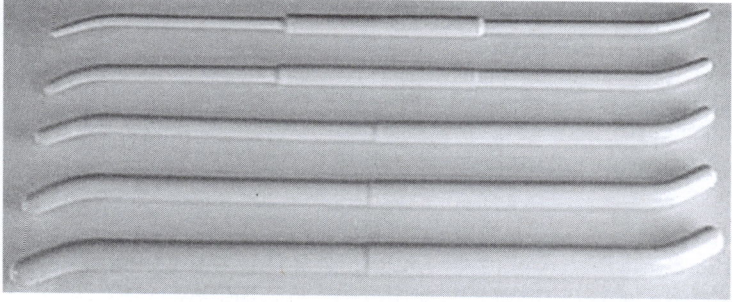

Fig. 32.16: Denniston dilators

INSTRUMENTS FOR CURETTING UTERINE CAVITY

1. Blunt and Sharp Curette

This is double-ended curette having one sharp end and the other blunt end. Sharp end is used for curetting endometrium from nonpregnant uterus while blunt end is used in postabortal/postpartum uterus to avoid injury to the soft uterus.

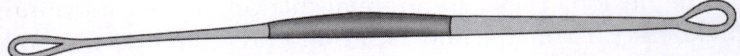

Fig. 32.17: Blunt and sharp curette

2. Novak's Endometrial Biopsy Curette

This slender instrument is used for obtaining a strip of endometrium for studying its hormonal status in cases like infertility, amenorrhoea or dysfunctional uterine bleeding. The instrument is slightly curved having a serrated eye at the tip. The curetted endometrial strip is collected by either pushing with a stylet or flushing with a syringe.

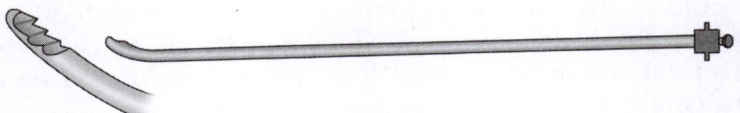

Fig. 32.18: Novak's endometrial biopsy curette

Advantage

Being a slender instrument of 4 mm diameter, cervical dilatation is not required; hence no anaesthesia is required.

Disadvantage

Pathological lesions like tuberculosis or malignancy may be patchy and hence are likely to be missed. For diagnosis of such conditions, thorough curettage is necessary.

Cervical Biopsy Punch

This stout instrument has a long handle and punch jaw. It is used for obtaining cervical biopsy. The biopsy piece is caught in its basket jaw.

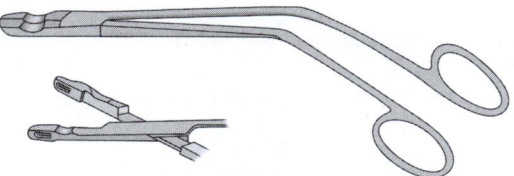

Fig. 32.19: Cervical biopsy punch

Ayre's Spatula

This wooden or plastic spatula is used for obtaining vaginal or cervical cellular material for cytological study. The conical part of the bifurcated end is inserted into cervical canal to scrape endocervical epithelium while the butt shapped end scrapes the ectocervical epithelium simultaneously. Since squamo-columnar junction is scraped completely, greater diagnostic accuracy is achieved. The spade shaped end is used to obtain vaginal cells by scraping lateral vaginal walls.

Cytobrush is used for obtaining sample from endocervical canal.

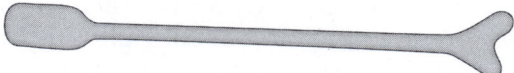

Fig. 32.20: Ayre's spatula

TUBAL PATENCY INSTRUMENTS

1. Rubin's Cannula

The cannula is long with a curved end to negotiate the uterine position. It has got an adjustable rubber or fixed metal cone, which fits snugly into the external cervical os.

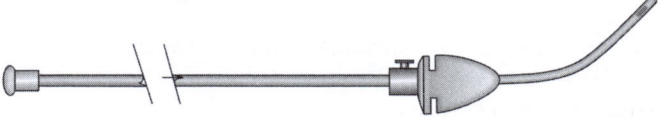

Fig. 32.21: Rubin's cannula

2. Leech-Wilkinson Cannula

This instrument is having a serrated cone near the tip to fit snugly into the external cervical os. These cannulae are used for testing tubal patency and for hydrotubation.

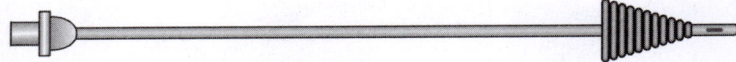

Fig. 32.22: Leech-Wilkinson cannula

3. Shirodkar's Isthmus Occluding Clamp

This is an instrument devised for testing tubal patency during laparotomy. Two curved sleeves at the lower end hold on the isthmus firmly to occlude it while the triangular space between the two shank accommodates the uterus.

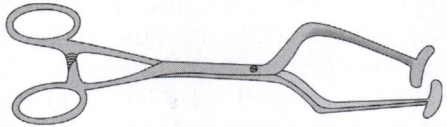

Fig. 32.23: Shirodkar's isthmus occluding clamp

Shirodkar's Ligature Carriers

This is a special curved needle with an eye at the tip and a long handle. They are used in pair, one for right side and one for the left. A small sized set is used for cervical encerclage by Shirodkar's technique while a large sized set is used for Shirodkar's posterior sling operation for correction of genital prolapse.

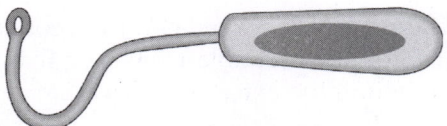

Fig. 32.24: Shirodkar's ligature carriers

ABDOMINAL RETRACTORS

1. Right-angled Retractor

It has got a small narrow rectangular blade at right-angle to the handle. It is useful for tubectomy by minilaparotomy. A larger size retractor with larger blade is used to retract urinary bladder in vaginal hysterectomy.

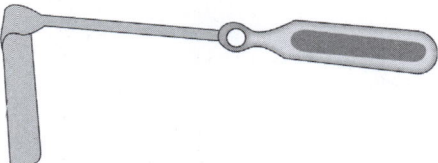

Fig. 32.25: Right-angled retractor

2. Deaver's Abdominal Retractors

They are provided with a long curved retracting blade. They are available in different sizes. This retractor gives a good exposure due to its curvature and is particularly useful in radical hysterectomy.

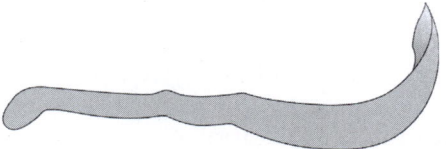

Fig. 32.26: Deaver's abdominal retractor

3. Doyen's Retractor

Due to the broad C shaped blade, it gives a good access to the uterovesical pouch by retracting the lower end of abdominal incision with the urinary bladder. It is used in lower segment caesarean section.

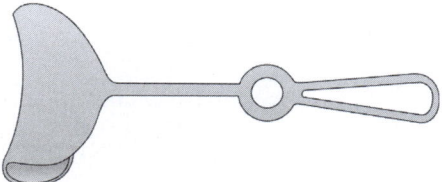

Fig. 32.27: Doyen's retractor

4. Self-retaining Retractor

The two lateral blades are mounted on a transverse bar. One blade is fixed while the other one is sliding. The third detachable

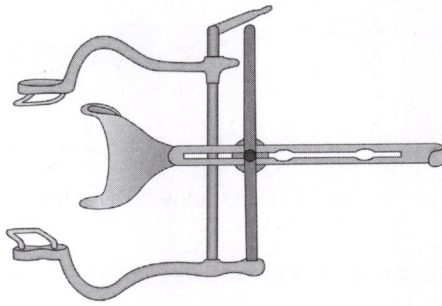

Fig. 32.28: Self-retaining retractor

blade retracts the lower end of the abdominal incision with urinary bladder and it can be fixed to the retractor by means of a screw. Due to its self-retaining property, one assistant can be spared. It gives a very good exposure.

Bonney's Myomectomy Clamp

The instrument was designed to minimise the bleeding during myomectomy by occluding the uterine arteries temporarily. Its sharply angulated strong and stout blade-shanks are covered with rubber tubes. It has two pairs of finger rings. It is applied from front to grip the body of the uterus just above the cervix. It must include both the round ligaments in its grip to prevent its slipping. It cannot be used in cases with large cervical or broad ligament fibroids.

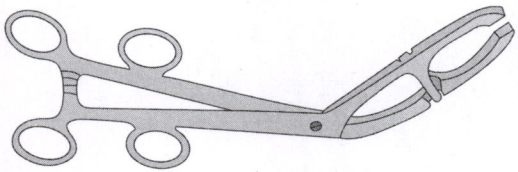

Fig. 32.29: Bonney's myomectomy clamp

Berkeley-Bonney Vaginal Clamp

This is a stout long instrument for clamping the vagina before opening it during Wertheim's radical hysterectomy, to avoid

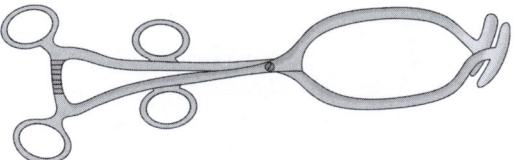

Fig. 32.30: Berkeley-Bonney vaginal clamp

spillage of malignant cells from the cervix into the vagina. The vagina is clamped by two serrated jaws provided at its terminal end and is cut below the clamp. Its shanks are bowed so as to include the uterus without compressing it. It is provided with two pairs of finger-rings, the lower one is used for adjustment, while the upper one is used while clamping the vagina. Being a large instrument, it is very difficult to manipulate, hence it may be substituted by strong clamps like Myxter forceps, curved on sides at right-angle for clamping the vagina.

INSTRUMENTS FOR HOLDING TISSUES

1. Kocher's Forceps

These are straight or curved stout tissue forceps and are provided with 1 × 2 teeth at their terminal ends. These teeth ensure a firm grip of the tissues or pedicles. They are used for clamping the ligaments during hysterectomy and grasping and crushing pedicles of tumours and cysts.

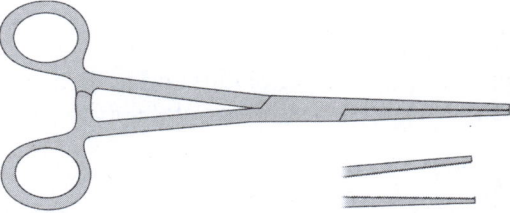

Fig. 32.31: Kocher's forceps

2. Allis Tissue Forceps

These are straight forceps with L shaped tips at the terminal end. Comparatively, it is a less traumatizing instrument. They are available in different sizes.

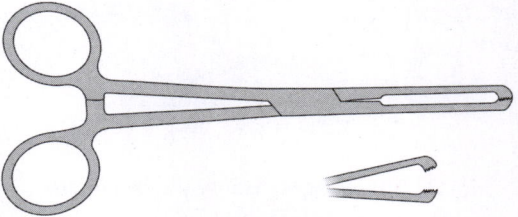

Fig. 32.32: Allis tissue forceps

3. Babcock's Tissue Forceps

They are having rounded serrated fenestrated and nontraumatic ends. They are very delicate. They are used to hold delicate tubular structures like fallopian tubes, ureters, appendix, etc. They are commonly used in tubectomy operation.

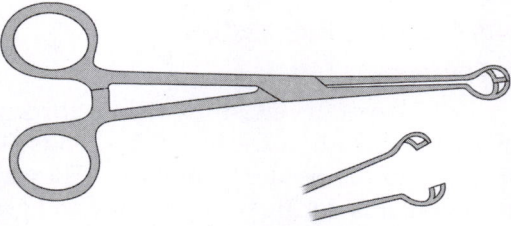

Fig. 32.33: Babcock's tissue forceps

4. Green-Armytage Forceps

These forceps have triangular blades and a catch at the handles. The base of the triangle has horizontal serrations. They are 8

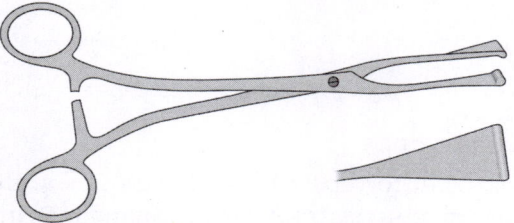

Fig. 32.34: Green-Armytage forceps

inches in length. They are used to catch the edges of uterine incision during caesarean section. They control the bleeding from uterine edges by compression without damaging.

5. Ovum Forceps

This tissue forceps is without a catch at the handle. It has spoon shaped fenestrated blades at the terminal end of the long shanks to catch the products of conception during evacuation of the uterus. The products are caught and the forceps are rotated around itself before bringing out. Thus if uterine wall is caught accidently, it slips as there is no catch.

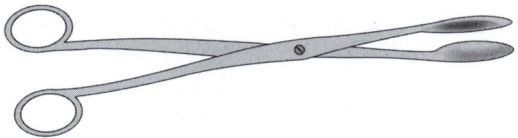

Fig. 32.35: Ovum forceps

Use

To evacuate the uterus of the products of conception, placental bits or molar tissue.

SCISSORS

1. Episiotomy Scissors

This is a pair or scissors, sharply angulated on the side at the joint. They are designed to give episiotomy.

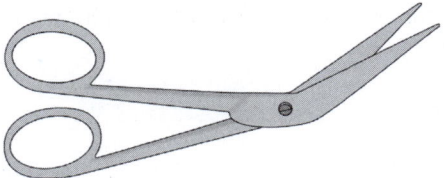

Fig. 32.36: Episiotomy scissors

2. Umbilical Cord Scissors

This is a pair of scissors having short circular blades, which give a good grip to the slippery cord.

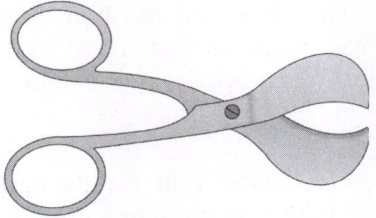

Fig. 32.37: Umbilical cord scissors

BLADDER CATHETERS

1. Metal Catheter

Female metal catheter is shorter in length than male metal catheter as the female urethra is shorter in length. It is used for draining the bladder during vaginal surgery. It is not used during labour as it can cause trauma and can lead to a false passage.

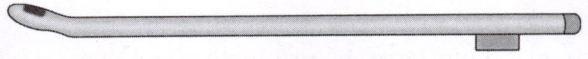

Fig. 32.38: Metal catheter

2. Flexible Catheters

Simple Catheter

It can be rubber or polythene catheter. It is a simple hollow tube with eyes at two sides at its closed tip to drain urine.

In cases of prolonged labour with deeply engaged head, the patient is unable to empty her bladder when catheterization is

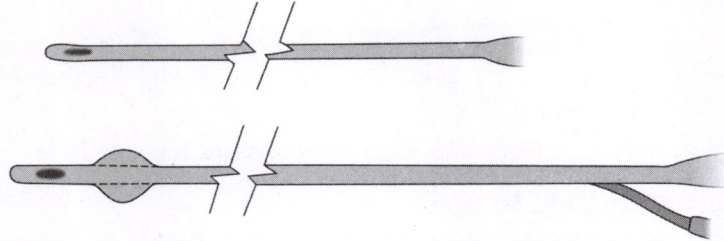

Fig. 32.39: Flexible catheters. 1. Simple rubber catheter; 2. Foley's catheter

required. Passage of rubber catheter is at times difficult due to compression of urethra. Forcible introduction of metal catheter can lead to a false passage; hence should be strictly avoided. Instead, introduction of two fingers vaginally between the head and the urethra can allow the passage of a flexible catheter.

Self-retaining Catheters

They are used for continuous drainage of the bladder, avoiding the need for repeated catheterization.

Uses in Gynaecology

During immediate postoperative period: Anterior colporrhaphy (48 hours), radical hysterectomy (10 days), repaired bladder injury (7–10 days), vesicovaginal fistula repair (21 days).

Uses in Obstetrics

a. Unconcious patients, e.g. in eclampsia.
b. Acute retention of urine due to retroverted gravid uterus impacted in pelvis.
c. Postoperatively after caesarean section performed for obstructed labour with threatened or actual uterine rupture with haematuria.
d. To minimise the risk of fistula formation due to prolonged compression of urinary bladder in prolonged obstructed labour due to deep transverse arrest.

Foley's Catheter

These are latex rubber catheters having two channels – one for draining urine and the other for instilling saline to inflate the bulb provided near the tip to retain the catheter. The capacity of the bulb is 30 ml. The bulb is deflated, before removal.

Other Uses of Foley's Catheter

a. Extra-amniotic instillation of ethacridine lactate for second trimester MTP.

b. Pre-induction ripening of the cervix in cases having poor Bishop's score and for induction of labor

c. Prevent reformation of intrauterine synechae after their lysis-paediatric Foley's catheter is used.

d. Intraoperative tubal patency test by keeping the catheter into the uterine cavity to occlude the internal os.

e. For diagnosis of incompetent internal os of cervix.

f. During cervical encerclage, for reducing and protecting the bulging bag of membranes in advanced cases of cervical incompetence. For this use, tip of the catheter is cut and only the bulb is used.

Index

Abdominal hysterectomy 56
Abdominal hysterotomy 207
Abdominal retractors 354
Absolute contraindications 224
Actinomycin D 326
Actions of forceps 137
Active immunization against
    hepatitis B 304
Adenocarcinoma of endocervix 26
Admission register 187
Advantages of lower segment
    caesarean section 160
Alendronate 324
Allis tissue forceps 357
Alpha methyl dopa 284
Amniocentesis 114
Analgesics 307
Anterior
    cervical myoma 77
    colporrhaphy 83
Anticoagulant drugs 305
Anticonvulsant drugs in
    eclampsia 287
Anti-d immunoglobulin 306
Antidote 306
Antifertility effects of prolactin 211
Antifungal agents 310
Antihypertensive drugs 284
Anti-hypertensive drugs not recomm-
    ended during pregnancy 286
Antiretroviral therapy (ART) during
    pregnancy 328
Architectural and cytologic
    features 10
Aspirin 290
Atenelol 286
Atociban 303
Authorization of the medical
    specialists 122

Auvard's speculum 344
Axis-traction 144
Ayre's spatula 353

Babcock's tissue forceps 358
Barrier devices for females 215
Basal body temperature (BBT)
    method 209
Beneficial effects 225
Berkeley-bonney vaginal clamp 356
Bethesda system (2001) 15
Bird's cup 148
Bladder catheters 360
Bladder
    injury 92
    sound 350
Blades 145
Blunt and sharp curette 352
B-lynch suture 172
Bonney's myomectomy clamp 356
Broad ligament myoma 77
Bromocriptine 316
B–sympathomimetic drugs 298

Cabergoline 317
Carboprost tromethamine (15
    methyl PGF_2-α) 294
Care of device 219
Causes of
    non-response 282
    retension 180
Cauterization 28
Caution while oral contraceptive
    use 224
Cellular criteria suggesting
    malignancy 14
Central cervical myoma 77

363

Cervical
  biopsy 19
    punch 352
  caps 218
  fibroids 76
  incompetence 203
  intraepithelial neoplasia (CIN) 12
  lacerations 201
  secretions to identify fertile period (billing's method) 210
Cetrorelix (GNRH antagonist) 320
Characteristics 145
Check points for correct vacuum extractor placement 150
Chemical sterilization 264
Chemotherapy in gynaecological malignancies 325
Cherney incision 341
CHO multiple square compression sutures 173
Choice of drug 298
Chorion villus biopsy 117
Cisplatinum 327
Classical caesarean section 164
Cleidotomy 179
Clomiphene + dexamethazone 315
Clomiphene + HCG 315
Clomiphene + oestrogen 315
Clomiphene citrate 313
Closure of abdomen 341
CO_2 laser therapy 31
Colposcopic findings 18
Colposcopy 16
Colposcopy in therapy 18
Combined oral contraceptive pills 222
Combined spinal epidural anesthesia 158
Complications of
  abdominal tubectomy 258
  fistula repair 91
  MRP 181
  surgical procedures of first trimester MTP 199

Components of malstrom vacuum extractor 148
Composition of different pills 223
Comyns-berkeley's vulval retractor 346
Condoms 213
Cone biopsy 22
Consent for MTP 187
Conservative surgical procedures for management of PPH 170
Contraception after vasectomy 273
Contraceptive
  benefits 232
  patch 235
  sponge 220
  vaginal ring (nuvaring) 233
Copper-T200 239
Cordocentesis (foetal blood sampling) 118
Cornual implantation 44
Correction of anaemia 281
Corticosteroids 304
Counseling 268
  points 254
Craniotomy 175
Creation of artificial vagina 95
Criteria for the correct application of blades 140
Criteria to be fulfilled before application of forceps 138
Cryotherapy 29
Cusco's bivalve self-retaining vaginal speculum 344
Cyclophosphamide 327
Cytology screening 15

Danazol 312
Deaver's abdominal retractors 355
Decapitation 177
Degrees 133
Denniston dilators 351
Detrusor overactivity 85

Diagnosis
   during pregnancy 105
   tests and preoperative
      evaluation 88
Diazepam 289
Difficulties 252
   in forceps delivery 142
Dilatation and
   curettage 4
   evacuation 198
Dinoprostone 295
Dinoprostone gel 295
Directed biopsy 19
Diuretics 287
Dose of the ethacridine lactate 204
Doyen's retractor 355
Drug combination 290
Drug of choice 287
Drugs 311
Drugs suggested 284

Effects of oral iron 281
Electrical vacuum aspiration
   (suction evacuation) 196
Electrocautery 28
Electrocoagulation diathermy 28
Emergency contraception 235
Endometrial biopsy 4
Endometrial hyperplasia 10
Epidural 158
Episiotomy scissors 359
Estrogen + progestin combined
   injectables 233
Evisceration 178
Exfoliative cytology 13
Extent of hysterectomy 170
External cephalic version 125
Extra-amniotic instillation of
   ethacridine lactate 203
Extra-amniotic methods 203
Extraction of head 146

Failed forceps 143
Female condom 216

Fenton's dilators 351
Fertility awareness based
   methods 208
Fimbrioplasty 42
Fixing and staining of smears 14
Flexible catheters 360
Foetal tissue biopsy 120
Foetoscopy 118
Folic acid 284
For induction/augmentation of
   labour 291
Fothergill's (manchester)
   operation 67
Fractional curettage 6

Genetic centers 120
Genuine stress incontinence 81
Gestational trophoblastic
   diseases 325
Gestrinone 312
GNRH agonists depot forms:
   triptorelin (decapeptyl) 319
GNRH analogues (GNRHA) 318
GNRHA triptorelin 312
Gonadotropins 317
Green-Armytage forceps 358

Haemorrhage 202
Hegar's dilators 350
Heparin 305
Hepatitis B immunoglobin
   (HBIG) 304
Hirsutism 325
Historical 152
Hormone replacement therapy
   (HRT) for menopause 323
Hormones 320
Hysterosalpingography 33
Hysteroscopic sterilization 263
Hysteroscopy 50

Immediate postoperative
   period 259
Indications for dilatation only 4

Indications for endometrial
   curettage 3
Indications for removal of IUD 252
Indomethacin 302
Induction of ovulation 313, 314
Induction–abortion interval 205
Inevitable and incomplete
   abortions 101
Infection 202
Information obtained by cervical
   biopsy 21
Information to patients 191
Informed consent 254
Inhibitory drugs could be
   potentially harmful 298
Initial treatment 89
Injectable contraception progestin
   only injectables 231
Injuries to ureter 93
Injury recognized during surgery 93
Injury recognized late 94
Instructions for BOM 210
Instructions to the patient 30
Instruments
   for curetting uterine cavity 352
   for dilating cervix 350
   for grasping and steadying
      cervix 346
   for holding tissues 357
   used for disinfecting the parts 348
Internal podalic version 128
Interval sterilization by
   minilaparotomy 257
Interval tubectomy 254
Intrauterine synaechiae 203
Intravenous pyelography 89
Iron dextran (imferon) 282
Iron sorbitol citric acid complex
   (jectofer) 283
Iron sucrose 282

Jayle's vaginal retractor 346
Joel cohen incision 340

Kjelland's forceps 145
Kleihauer test 307
Kocher's forceps 357

Labetelol 286
Labetelol IV (avoid in asthma) 286
Lactational amenorrhoea
   method 211
Laparoscopic
   chromotubation 36
   hysterectomy 49
   multiple punctures of the cysts
      with electrocautery or laser 79
   sterilization 260
Laparoscopy 45
Lateral cervical myoma 77
LAVH 49
LAVH (laparoscopic assisted
   vaginal hysterectomy) 49
Layers incised in episiotomy 131
Le Fort's operation (colpocleisis) 71
Leech-Wilkinson cannula 353
Levels of forceps 136
Ligation of internal iliac artery 170
Light amplification by stimulated
   emission of radiation 31
Limitations of colposcopy 18
LNG IUS 312
Loop electrosurgical excision
   procedure (LEEP) 21
Lower segment caesarean
   section 159
Lytic cocktail 290

Magnesium sulfate 287, 301
Malignant potential of different
   types 10
Management guidelines for
   endometrial cancer 7
Management of uterine
   perforation 200
Manual vacuum aspiration
   (MVA) 193

Mayo-Ward's operation 66
McDonald's operation 106
McIndoe operation 95
Medical abortion 189
Medical fitness 255
Medical methods 205
Mefenamic acid (antipro-
staglandin) 311
Menorrhagia 311
Menstrual regulation 191
Metal catheter 360
Metformin 315
Methods for first trimester
MTP 189, 191
Methods for second trimester
MTP 189, 203
Methods of insertion 244
Methotrexate 326
Methyl ergometrine 293
Metoclopramide 309
Metronidazole 309
Metroplasty 96
Midurethral slings: tension free
vaginal tape (TVT) 85
Mifepristone 190
Minor side effects 226
Mirena intrauterine system 240
Misconceptions regarding
vasectomy 269
Misgav Ladach technique 162
Misoprostol 190
Missed
abortion 102
pill 229
Mityvac 147
Mode of administration 291
Modified burch colposus-
pension 83
Monthly report 188
Moschcowitz operation 70
Mould 95
Multiload Cu 250 and Cu 375 239

Nature of injury 93
Needle suspension procedures:
(Pareyra, Stamey) 85
Neonatal complications 151
Nifedipine 285, 301
Nimodipine 286
Nitroglycerin 302
No visceral injury 200
Non-contraceptive benefits 232
Nonhormonal therapy for
menopausal women 324
Non-steroidal oral pill:
centchroman 237
Nonsurgical management 111
Novak's endometrial biopsy
curette 352
Nutritional anaemia complicating
pregnancy 281

Obstetric forceps 135
Obstetric hysterectomy 169
Obtaining material for cytological
smears 13
Oestrogens 320
Offences and penalties 123
Oophorectomy 79
Operative principles 75
Opinion for performing MTP 187
Oral iron 281
Oral progestogens 311
Other use of MR syringe 193
Ovarian cancer 327
Ovarian cystectomy 78
Ovariotomy 78
Overflow incontinence 86
Ovum forceps 359
Oxytocic drugs 291
Oxytocin 291

Pajot's manoeuvre 144
Parenteral iron 282
Parts of obstetric forceps 136
Pentazocin (fortwin) 308

Perineal tears (irregular lacerations of perineum) 133
Pessary for correction of genital prolapse 72
Pethidine 307
Phenytoin sodium 289
Physiological principles 208
Place of ECV 128
Place of the preconceptional encerclage 111
Playfair's probe 349
Post conization hysterectomy 24
Post insertion instructions 246
Post-cauterization instructions 29
Posterior
   cervical myoma 77
   fundal implantation 44
PPTCT program 329
Preconceptional management 111
Preeclampsia–eclampsia 284
Prenatal diagnostic procedures 123
Prerequisites for use of tocolytic drugs 297
Prevention of
   hepatitis B 304
   Rh isoimmunization 306
Principle of surgery 257
Principles of microsurgery 41
Progesterones 322
Progestogen only pills: mini pills 230
Progestogens for use in gynaecologic conditions 322
Progestogens for use in pregnancy 322
Promethazine 308
Prophylactic premenopausal oophorectomy at hysterectomy 79
Prophylaxis of iron deficiency anaemia 281
Prostaglandins 294
Pudendal block 139

Puerperal tubectomy 253, 256
Pulsatile GnRH agonist therapy 319
Purandare's cervicopexy 70
Purandare's dilators 351
Purpose of dilatation and curettage 8

Raloxifene 325
Record maintenance 124
Registration of genetic centers 121
Relative contraindications 224
Removal of the stitch 107
Retroversion 73
Rhythm method (calendar method) 209
Right-angled retractor 354
Risk of
   bladder injury 92
   emergency contraception 236
Routes 53
   of administration 323
Routine vs selective episiotomy 133
Rubin's cannula 353

Safe forceps 142
Safety of ARV 331
Saline test 38
Salpingolysis and ovariolysis 42
Salpingostomy 43
Scissors 359
Secrecy 188
Selection of
   acceptors 224
   treatment modality 65
Selective β_2 agonists 300
Self-retaining retractor 355
Shirodkar's
   isthmus occluding clamp 354
   ligature carriers 354
   modification of Fothergill's operation 68

operation 108
posterior sling 69
Sialastic cup 147
Significance of abnormal cervical
    smear and suggested
    management 25
Sim's anterior vaginal wall
    retractor 345
Sim's speculum 343
Some common techniques 264
Some currently used devices 238
Sonosalpingography 37
Soonawala speculum 345
Sounds 349
Special preoperative
    preparations 102
Spinal anaesthesia 156
Spironolactone 325
Sponge holding forceps 347, 348
Stepwise uterine
    devascularization 174
Sterilization of IUD and
    inserter 244
Sterilization of the MR kit 192
Subsequent labour 134, 166
Subsequent pregnancy 76
Success of fistula repair 91
Success rate 205
Suprapubic sling operations 84
Surgical closure 89
Surgical technique 97, 256
Surgical treatment 81
Suturing 132
Symptoms 85
Symptothermal method 210

Techniques for preventing reunion
    of vas 274
Techniques of tubal oblitera-
    tion 264
Tenaculum forceps 347
Terratogenic drugs 332
The aims of surgery 83

The preconception and prenatal
    diagnostic techniques act
    2003 120
The prerequisites for MTP
    centre 186
Therapeutic amniocentesis 115
Therapeutic benefits of diagnostic
    tests 40
Therapeutic scope of
    foetoscopy 118
Therapeutic surgical 51
Tibolone 324
Tinidazole or secnidazole 310
Tocolytic drugs 296
Today vaginal contraceptive
    pessaries 219
Toxoplasmosis during preg-
    nancy 303
Transabdominal encerclage 110
Transdermal estrogen patch 324
Transperitoneal extravesical
    repair 90
Transverse incisions 339
Transverse muscle cutting incision
    (Maylard incision) 340
Transvesical repair 90
Treatment of endometriosis 312
Treatment of hyperstimulation 292
Trial forceps 143
Triple screen or multiple marker
    screen test 116
Tubal
    anastomosis 43
    block 203
    implantation 43
    patency instruments 353
Tubal patency tests 33
Tubal reconstructive surgery 40
Types of
    application of blades 136
    caesarean sections 153
    cervical biopsies 19
    implants 234

Ultrasonography 112
Umbilical cord scissors 359
Urinary fistulae 86
Urinary tract injuries (during
    gynaecological surgery) 91
Use for medical abortion 190
Use of pessary 111
Uterine
    perforation 199
    sound 349

Vacuum extractor (ventouse) 146
Vaginal diaphragm (dutch
    cap) 217
Vaginal
    hysterectomy 60
    repair 89
    speculae 343
    tubectomy 261

Vaginitis 309
Value of colposcopy 17
Vasectomy 268
Vertical incisions 338
Vertical uterine compression
    sutures 172
Vesicular mole 102
Video endoscopy 49
Visceral injury 201
Volsellum forceps 346

Weakness of classical scar on
    uterus 165
Wertheim's radical hysterec-
    tomy 59
William's vulvovaginoplasty 96
Withdrawal method (coitus
    interruptus) 212
Wurm procedure 110

Reader's Notes

Reader's Notes